How to Get Fit – and Stay Fit

Michael Blate is well known as a leading teacher and authority in the art (or science) of self-health. He has appeared on nationwide radio and television in Britain and the USA, and is the author of more than a dozen books in the field of natural health and healing without drugs or medicines, including *The Natural Healer's Acupressure Handbook: G-Jo Fingertip Technique*, *Advanced G-Jo*, *How to Heal Yourself Using Hand Acupressure*, *How to Heal Yourself Using Foot Acupressure*, and (with Gail Watson) *Cooking Naturally For Pleasure and Health*, all published by Routledge & Kegan Paul.

How to Get Fit – and Stay Fit

The Acugenic Method

Michael Blate
with Gail C. Watson, M.S.

ARKANA

London, Melbourne and Henley

First published in 1985
by ARKANA PAPERBACKS
ARKANA PAPERBACKS is an imprint of
Routledge & Kegan Paul plc

14 Leicester Square, London WC2H 7PH, England

464 St Kilda Road, Melbourne,
Victoria 3004, Australia and

Broadway House, Newtown Road,
Henley-on-Thames, Oxon RG9 1EN, England

Typset by Columns, Reading
Printed and bound in Great Britain by
The Guernsey Press Co Ltd,
Guernsey, Channel Islands

ISBN 1-85063-009-7

This book is for Keith . . .

Contents

Acknowledgments

For all the information from teachers and authors about acupuncture and acupressure techniques, this author extends his sincerest appreciation. While many have contributed to the dissemination of information about these traditionally Oriental self-health methods, the reader is advised to see publications by the American authors: Dr Ralph A. Dale (The Acupuncture Education Center, Miami, Florida); Dr Pedro Chan (Center for Chinese Medicine, Monterey Park, California 91754); Dr Robert E. Willner, M.D. (North Miami Beach, Florida 33165); Dr John Thie, D.C. (Touch for Health Foundation, Pasadena, California); and numerous other popular author-teachers of these techniques.

In Great Britain, Dr J.R. Worsley and Dr Felix Mann have been at the forefront of acupuncture education, and the authors Denis and Joyce Lawson-Wood have provided the public a great deal of useful self-health information. Their publications – as well as any other in the field of traditional Oriental self-applied health and healing techniques – are highly recommended.

And, finally, for her unceasing effort with this – and all other books in this series – this author extends his deepest thanks to Sandy Pasquale.

What is the G-Jo Institute?

The G-Jo Institute is a not-for-profit natural health research and educational organization. It was informally organized in 1976 and incorporated in 1982. Its purpose is the dissemination of drugless 'self-health' techniques.

G-Jo is a simplified form of acupuncture without needles (or 'acupressure'). However, the scope of the G-Jo Institute has expanded far beyond its original purpose of the sharing of simple acupressure techniques.

It is our belief that it is the body-mind – and *only* the body-mind – which heals itself. For that reason, we now address ourselves to the *entire* spectrum of how to stimulate the innate self-healing mechanisms within the body-mind with simple, yet effective, self-applied techniques from around the world.

For further information or catalogs about our publications, recordings, workshops and such, send a business-sized, self-addressed stamped envelope to:

THE G-JO INSTITUTE
DIVISION AF
POST OFFICE BOX 8060
HOLLYWOOD, FLA. 33024
U.S.A.

What is ACUGENICS?

'Acugenics' means *that which has its basis in the acupuncture (energy) theory*. This traditionally-Oriental viewpoint believes that a vital force – called *bioenergy* – circulates from organ to organ throughout the body, making them produce the chemicals and electromagnetic impulses vital for life.

When bioenergy is moving smoothly from organ to organ – neither too quickly nor too slowly – we are in good health. But when any disruption or malfunction occurs within the energy system, symptoms appear and we are considered to be ill. In this Oriental point of view, there are thousands of symptoms but only one disease: an 'imbalanced' flow of bioenergy.

The techniques and information in the following pages have a single purpose – to help the body-mind restore balance and harmony within its bioenergy system. As this occurs, the entire body-mind begins feeling better . . . excess weight is shed . . . and we gradually take on a more youthful and vital appearance. Our strength and stamina are increased and we become more limber and flexible. Emotional slumps become less traumatic and our outlook on life improves. In short, life becomes happier, healthier and, through the process, more rich and rewarding. Such is the power of Acugenics.

Foreword

Good health is life in motion. And being physically fit can be an affirmation that life in motion can be enjoyably expressed through a well-conditioned body. For some, physical fitness is measured by the number of miles run, laps swum, or pushups done. It is a quantity of energy or strength, directed toward some specific level of achievement. Being able to DO some measurable physical feat then becomes both the goal and the reward. And the achievement of a particular goal becomes a prime motivator.

Another way of looking at physical fitness is as a level of EXPERIENCE, a way of moving through one's life, a way of flowing. From this perspective, physical fitness is not so much a matter of bodily strength or achievement. Rather, it is a quality of aliveness, a measure of freedom. The Oriental Tai Chi master, for example, is physically fit, not in terms of where he can get to or how fast he can get there. His strength and fitness are grounded in flexibility, centeredness, and alertness. He is fit partly by virtue of where he can move in his CONSCIOUSNESS, in his inner awareness, in the very core of his being.

So, physical fitness, in the fullest sense, is not 'physical' at all. It is a dynamic state of aliveness rooted in the whole person. It is a quality of being balanced, flexible . . . response-able, if you will, to any assaults that may come forth. In life, we often spend a lot of our energy responding to and dealing with these assaults. Physical assaults, in which we may be challenged to defend ourselves or others from attack, are relatively rare. It is assaults upon other levels of our being, even some that come from within ourselves, that may continually occupy us . . . emotional assaults (for example, harsh criticism from boss, spouse, athletic trainer, etc.), mental assaults (for example, the worries and fears that we ourselves generate through our imaginings of unwanted outcomes), even spiritual assaults, by leaving ourselves too wide open at times to the harsh vibrations of others around us. True physical fitness can help us respond to these challenges in a way that will keep us protected from injury or harm.

So, physical fitness becomes a matter of training, not only of training the body, but of restructuring thoughts and emotions, as well. Motivation is required to break out of old limitations. And the discipline of repetition is needed to reacquaint the body-mind with its innate ability to flow in harmony with its surroundings.

Part of the message of this book is that you can be GENTLE with yourself. Harsh exercise, stringent schedules and routines, and heroic levels of achievement are not encouraged, or even recommended. What you ARE encouraged to do is to move . . . in your physical body, in your consciousness, in your mental and emotional patterns, toward a more fluid way of being-in-the-world. This is a guidebook that will help you STRETCH . . . not only your muscles, but in your ability to enjoy, to the depths of your being, your interaction with all of life. Go ahead . . . REACH OUT!!!

Section I:
A Philosophy of Fitness

CAUTION: BEFORE UNDERTAKING THIS – OR ANY OTHER – FITNESS PROGRAM, PLEASE CHECK WITH YOUR DOCTOR OR HEALTH CARE PROFESSIONAL FIRST . . . ESPECIALLY IF YOU SUFFER FROM SEVERE, CHRONIC, OR DEBILITATING ILLNESS.

THE G-JO INSTITUTE ACUGENICS FITNESS PROGRAM is an easy-to-follow method of improving fitness and health for people of *all* ages and in nearly any state of health. It takes only 15 or 20 minutes to perform all the techniques you'll find in Section II of this manual; and in many cases you can easily abbreviate them to take less than 5 minutes to perform. But it is strongly suggested you read this section first.

ACUGENICS is an exciting concept which draws from the time-tested methods from the Orient (especially India, Tibet and China) as well as more conventional Western techniques. In the following pages is detailed a program that is easy, fun and (perhaps most important) *sustainable* for the rest of your life.

You don't have to run – or do other harsh, violent calisthenic-type exercises – to be healthy. In fact, there is every indication that harsh exercise can actually lead to *un*health and physical injury. Fitness – that is, having the strength, endurance, coordination and flexibility to do those things in your life which please you – comes from an on-going 'healthstyle', in which harsh exercise need never play a part.

The Test of Fitness

How do you know if you're really fit? There are simple guidelines and measurements you can use to determine your own level of fitness (and by knowing this, some reasonable goals to set that you'd like to achieve):

* Do you have enough energy to enjoy your life? (The fit and healthy person exudes a sense of glowing, dynamic energy and is able to lead as complete a life as he or she chooses – both for work and play);
* Do you suffer from chronic illness? (The fit, healthy person, while not necessarily free of all ailments, suffers physically and emotionally only for relatively short periods of time. Most acute illness is more a 'healing crisis', or throwing off of the accumulations from an abusive lifestyle – but longstanding or chronic problems reflect an ignorant way of living, wherein the sufferer has failed to learn the vital lessons that illness has to offer);
* Can you do the things you'd really *like* to do? (A healthy, fit person feels enthusiastic and confident – both about doing those things which he knows as well as attempting new activities and projects);
* Do you look and feel younger than you actually are? (The healthy, fit person has a youthful twinkle in his eyes and radiates a boundless sense of life and vitality, no matter what his age);

* Can you relax as well as work? (Proper relaxation is probably the single most important aspect of fitness – you'll see why later);
* Is your 'happiness level' at least 57 minutes of each hour? (The healthy – truly healthy – person is happy virtually all the time. If you find yourself less than pleased with being alive more than 3 minutes each hour your level of health and fitness still leaves something to be desired).

Fitness isn't only measured by feats of strength or endurance – it is a measure of comparison of how good you feel and look *now* versus how you *used to* feel and/or how good you *can* feel in the foreseeable future.

Fitness and Energy

The goal of this G-JO INSTITUTE ACUGENICS PROGRAM is ultimately to help you 'balance your energy'. Vital energy – which the Japanese call *ki* and the Chinese call *ch'i* – is the secret of fitness and health. This 'lifeforce' (which we can call *bioenergy*) travels along pathways, or 'meridians', of energy to and from the various organs and glands within the body.

When bioenergy is flowing properly – that is, neither too quickly nor too slowly along these meridians – our organs and glands function as they are supposed to. Then the body (and mind, rather the 'body-mind') is truly healthy and fit.

But if energy flow becomes disturbed (caused by, for example, wrong food, wrong emotions, wrong work, etc.), the organs and glands 'malfunction' and produce electrochemical chaos within the body-mind. When *that* occurs, health disorders and symptoms of deterioration begin manifesting themselves.

In the Orient it is said that there are thousands of symptoms but only one true disease: an imbalanced flow of energy. So 'poor fitness' – a very common group or syndrome of symptoms – is really an expression of imbalance within the electro-chemical system that links organs and glands with each other. Its symptoms often include flabbiness and poor muscle tone, low energy, being overweight, feeling older than our age and being unable to 'compete', etc.

Health is a physical *and* emotional or mental state of being. If fitness is only one aspect of good health, it is perhaps the most important one and without it, true health is not possible.

Fitness and Weight

For many people, being slender is synonymous with being healthy, while being even slightly overweight is synonymous with being unhealthy. Yet even slender people suffer from poor muscle tone, heart attacks, high blood pressure, diabetes, etc. . . . while *slightly* overweight (maximum of 5% above 'ideal' body weight) people tend to be the happiest individuals and live the longest.

Thus, weight is not necessarily the most important factor in fitness, even though they are commonly associated. While obese people can never be fit in the truest sense of the word, being slightly overweight is no hindrance in attaining a state of glowing well-being. However, you're too fat if you *feel* too fat – and this will interfere with any true feelings of fitness. So, if you feel you need to lose weight, by all means do it (a remarkably simple, yet effective way of losing excess weight is described in HOW TO LOSE WEIGHT EASILY: THE AUGENIC METHOD, from the same publishers).

A Main Obstacle to Fitness

While there is no single key to fitness, there *is* one problem which is most responsible for poor health, low energy and a generally unfit way of feeling: stress. Stress and tension – which appear to be at the root of more than three quarters of the illnesses suffered by modern man – have numerous negative effects on the body-mind.

Stress is a kind of low-level fear reaction (the so-called 'fight-or-flight' mechanism) which is 'stuck at half-cock'. This real or imagined sense of subtle threat eventually pervades the entire system and keeps the sufferer in a state of readiness to 'fight or flee'. For most people, this is a chronic state and one which affects them without actually reaching the conscious level of awareness except for brief periods.

It is safe to say that anyone who lives the 'normal' (Western) lifestyle – reading newspapers, watching television, working at a competitive job, raising a family, etc. – is suffering stress to a greater or lesser degree. This is particularly true for anyone eating 'normally' – that is, eating the typical diet rich in meat (*any* slaughtered food), salt, sugary or sweet foods and beverages, and 'convenience' foods. Right or wrong diet is perhaps the single most important key to stress or health and fitness (see below).

Stress deforms the body and keep at least some – and often many – of the muscles knotted and in a state of tension. Stress prevents coordination and harmony within; it destroys peace within the mind, emotions and spirit. And since inner peace is a fundamental element in fitness and health, the connection becomes easier to see.

Thus, a most important part of any fitness program is to first locate – then deal with – sources of stress and tension within your life. This may mean a job change, a new (and better) way of relating to the family or especially some important improvements in diet, as will be discussed shortly.

Why be Fit?

Most people live relatively comfortable and complacent lives until a traumatic experience jars them into looking at themselves and their healthstyles. The untimely death of a friend or family member . . . a sudden sense of aging or an unexpected illness . . . a recent divorce (or new love in one's life) – these are common reasons why people suddenly decide to become fit after years of living 'the good life'.

But any fitness program which is based on fear or panic – which many popular fitness programs are – tends to be too difficult to maintain for a meaningful length of time (namely, for one's whole life). Such programs – which usually require harsh exercise – fall easily by the wayside when the protective mechanism of the mind – called *homeostatis*, the protective reaction to sudden change – lures one back into old, comfortable habits.

Thus, a fitness program which fails to keep this 'rubber-band' effect in mind is eventually doomed to failure. Since ACUGENICS is a gentle program that also incorporates a number of mind-improving techniques, it is easy to maintain – or *return* to, should you occasionally 'forget'.

Factors Controlling Health and Fitness

Before describing The G-JO INSTITUTE ACUGENICS

FITNESS PROGRAM in detail, it is important to have a brief understanding of the factors that make up health (and which subsequently determine a reasonable – and *maintainable* – level of fitness for you). There are at least four important factors that must be considered, which include:

HEREDITY;
ENVIRONMENT;
ATTITUDE;
DIET.

Heredity

Of all the factors that influence health, nothing is more important than one's inherited, genetic constitution. While it is possible to 'rearrange' or 'remake' parts of one's basic body build, it is a difficult chore and requires an intense commitment to wellness. Fortunately, most people have relatively good constitutions; nature has a way of somehow eliminating the very weak or sickly.

Our genetic 'timeclocks' determine, more or less, the speed and degree of our aging as well as the weaknesses and infirmities we are likely to suffer during our lifetimes. Even with the best of preventive healthcare and maintenance, we are still partial prisoners of our hereditary constitutions (or, as a traditional Oriental doctor/philosopher might say, we are prisoners of our 'karma').

It is a rule of thumb that, the better your inherited constitution, the less difficult it is to achieve and maintain fitness; but the worse your hereditary constitution, the harder it is to stay fit and healthy. Improving one's inherited constitution usually requires techniques such as meditation and other 'psycho-physical' methods, as well as careful dietary controls throughout one's life.

As we age it is normal for changes – some of them rather surprising – to occur. For example: an older person generally needs less sleep or food than when he was younger; an older person is generally more coordinated than when he was younger; and an older person – especially one in good health – often has better endurance for certain activities than when he was a young person.

Thus, aging makes it easier, in many ways, to stay well and fit, especially if we have lived moderately in our early years.

Environment

Where and how we live – our homelife, our work and the geographical climate in which we live – are easier to change than our inherited constitutions but often such changes still create great obstacles to our wellness. For instance, we may know that our job is causing us stress, but either because we have no training or cannot afford the cut in pay that a new job might require, we find ourselves trapped into an unhealthy 'workstyle' whose primary (perhaps *only*) benefit is its paycheck. The same thing holds true for an inhospitable, but somehow convenient, love relationship, homelife or meteorological climate.

Staying fit and healthy is a life-long commitment. It is easy to become seduced and trapped into gradually forgetting that commitment as 'the good life' (or simply inertia) makes deeper and deeper inroads into health, vitality and energy. Also, staying well and fit requires a supportive environment: if our families fail to encourage us, then it is difficult to generate enough enthusiasm to continue *any* fitness program, even the least taxing. Thus, the *best* fitness program includes the whole family.

So without the right environment, not only is

maintaining fitness difficult, but even generating enough enthusiasm to *begin* such a program is hard. On the other hand, with a good environment, not only is attaining fitness much easier, but *maintaining* the simple routines in this program will become a fun and natural practice that lasts throughout life.

Attitude

How you feel about yourself and your life determines greatly what happens to your body and inner organs. Poor attitude and lack of fitness is like a dog chasing its tail: the less you like yourself or your surroundings, the harder it is to generate the enthusiasm needed for a successful fitness program; and the less fit you feel yourself to be, the more difficult it is to develop any strong feelings of self-worth.

On the other hand, fit people generally feel more alert and alive, which helps perpetuate the habits of life-long fitness.

Fortunately, attitude is more easily changed than heredity or environment: we may take classes, workshops or join wellness groups to accomplish this. Furthermore, the necessary attitudinal changes often occur about the same time that one decides to restore one's own health. In following this G-JO INSTITUTE ACUGENICS PROGRAM – because of its ease for people of all ages – there should be little, if any, problem in (re)establishing the right attitudes and habits for making these techniques a regular part of your own healthstyle for life.

Diet

Not only is the way that we eat the most easily changed of all the vital factors of fitness, but diet is so important that *with* right eating, little more needs to be done; and *without* it, nothing meaningful or permanent appears able to be done (in terms of life-long fitness).

Many people believe that exercise is the key to fitness: it is not. An animal – say, a cat – that eats moderately, has virtually no need to exercise (more than occasionally stretching and walking) to stay in good shape throughout its life. The human animal, too, has the same capabilities. Eating lightly-to-moderately is the surest way to stay fit and healthy. And keeping several important natural rules in mind when selecting food practically *guarantees* fitness and health.

How to Eat Best for Fitness and Health

First, *eat regionally and seasonally*: base your diet on *fresh* foods grown within 50 miles of your home (same environment). Avoid canned, processed or convenience food, selecting instead 'whole' foods (especially whole grains and vegetables – not refined, pre-prepared or commercially preserved, since each part of the food plays a vital role in its proper assimilation).

Next, move as quickly as possible to eating a *lacto-vegetarian diet*, using whole (brown) rice (and other complete grains) as the staple in your diet. Learn *food combining* – a method for mixing grains, legumes, dairy products, and such, for complete protein (see COOKING NATURALLY FOR PLEASURE AND HEALTH: A WAY OF EATING, by Gail C. Watson and Michael Blate, from the same publisher). Furthermore, the excess use of *any* dairy product should be dropped as soon as it is convenient. Dairy products are best used as 'bridge' foods between a meat-based and a slaughterless diet.

A vegetarian diet makes one feel lighter, more

energetic, 'cleaner' within and radiantly healthy – especially after the first several months of moving away from a meat-based diet (including *any* slaughtered product, even seafood or poultry). The fact that numerous athletes and sports personalities are turning/have turned to the vegetarian way of eating should be proof enough of its effectiveness.

Avoid abusive and allergenic foods or other consumables: if stress and tension are at the root of most illness, then 'wrong' foods – meaning those which produce a 'hidden' allergic reaction – are a prime cause of most stress and tension (a more complete discussion of this fascinating subject of hidden allergic reactions and their detection may be found in HOW TO LOSE WEIGHT EASILY: THE ACUGENIC METHOD).

Finally, sugar (or *any* harshly sweet food or drink), as well as alcohol, tobacco, caffeinated beverages, and even excessive medication – all of which affect the digestive organs badly – should be eliminated as quickly as possible. This is especially true if you drop slaughtered products from your diet. Sugar, alcohol and tobacco help boost the digestive organs to assimilate heavy meat products. But without meat to 'work on', sugary substances can cause depression, anger and other extreme emotions – all symptoms of the *liver* in distress, according to Oriental doctor-philosophers.

As a person moves away from unhealthy foods, his attitude gradually-to-quickly changes, especially if he drops slaughtered products, sweets, caffeine and alcohol from his life. And as his attitude changes, obstacles within his environment begin shrinking. Soon, the entire body-mind is feeling better and better.

Foods should be consumed in five or six smaller meals throughout the day, rather than two or three larger meals. Largest meals should be consumed earlier in the day with lighter meals taken in the late afternoon or evening. Select daily meals that are drawn from four basic food groups:

* *the milk group* (include at least two servings daily – assuming no dairy allergy exists – of milk, yogurt, *rennetless* cheese, etc.);
* *the protein group* (include at least two servings daily of beans, peas, lentils, nuts, tofu or other soy-bean products, etc.);
* *the grain/cereal group* (include at least four servings daily of whole, brown rice, whole wheat, pasta, etc.);
* *the fruit/vegetable group* (include at least four servings daily of any fresh fruit or vegetable in moderate amounts, in either whole or juice form).

In Section IV of this manual, you will find a selection of healthful, delicious recipes whose focus in on complete protein as well as 'quick energy' foods. More recipes, plus much useful information, is found in COOKING NATURALLY FOR PLEASURE AND HEALTH: A WAY OF EATING.

Abuse Destroys Health and Fitness

Abuse of any sort – especially smoking, excessive use of alcohol and abusive eating – is the main obstacle to, and destroyer of, health and fitness. No wellness program can truly compensate for the physical and emotional decay that such abusive practices cause. There are two vital rules to keep in mind when starting on any fitness/ wellness program:

* To get well and fit *you* must first *want* to get healthy (you can't do it 'because my wife wants me to' or 'my doctor said I should');

* To improve health and fitness you must *stop* the practices that *destroy* health.

The body-mind is a self-healing 'mechanism' that operates best when we are doing nothing to interfere with this ongoing process of self-healing. For example, sleep – probably the best healing technique of all – requires nothing from us except letting it happen. Thus, the fastest way to return to health – and to subsequent fitness – is by stopping the abuses that destroy us.

The primary abuse that most of us suffer is *putting too much (of anything) into our mouths*. Food . . . tobacco . . . excessive or wrong beverages . . . drugs – in other words, it is what we eat (consume by mouth) that injures us most. So the key to attaining/maintaining fitness and health, of course, is: *eat moderately, properly and humanely* (based on the rules described above).

The Role of Exercise, Health and Fitness

'Exercise' essentially means the *movement* (or *attempting the movement*) of something, say a heavy object. While no fitness program can be complete without some form of exercise, most of the movement we need is readily accomplished by slightly modifying the simple, everyday activities that most of us perform.

As you'll see below, walking as little as three or four hundred steps a day – which most of us do without thinking about it – provides enough movement and exercise to keep the muscles flexible and strong and even maintain our cardiovascular (blood and circulatory system) health . . . if our eating is right and we add the Acugenics energy-balancing methods.

Exercise – or movement – provides at least several vital services to the body-mind:

* It keeps muscles flexible . . .
* It frees lactic acid (and other 'tiredness chemicals' – those produced from stress, etc.) from the muscles to freshen us . . .
* It keeps the cardiovascular system operating normally (especially important if you are eating slaughtered foods or less-than-ideally) . . .
* And – most important – *it helps keep bioenergy moving properly along its meridians* (remember: when energy moves properly from organ to organ, you feel good physically *and* emotionally – you are fit and healthy).

Why Some People Need Harsh Exercise

Much of the need to run and do other violent exercises comes from a diet that is high in sugar and/or slaughtered products. 'Extreme foods' such as these create stress and tension, which in turn call for harsh exercise or activity to 'drain' or 'burn' the stress. The more animal protein or stress-producing foods we consume, the more necessary becomes harsh or violent activity to restore balance and harmony within.

Eliminating meat, alcohol, medicinal or 'recreational' drugs, harsh sweets and most salt from the diet eliminates much of the need – and much of the *desire* – for harsh exercise, such as running, tennis, etc. *Simple, gentle* exercise is the most natural and complete of all therapies. Its function is to increase the circulation and flow of vital bioenergy and to restore electro-chemical balance within the organs, the glands and muscles.

All movement (exercise) has the same effect but in varying degrees: it 'opens' and relaxes the meridians of energy, bringing tone and flexibility to the entire body-mind. (The existence of these energy pathways – which tend to parallel nerve channels – has now been clearly proven by Western science.) But any exercise, movement or activity that the body-mind tends to rebel against – such as any prolonged, harsh exercise program – is the system's statement that, while one organ or gland may be receiving a benefit, numerous others are suffering.

Nowhere is this better illustrated than with running: while the cardiovascular system may receive some temporary benefits (which are lost within a few days after a running program stops), the genito-urinary system (the kidneys, urinary bladder, etc.) as well as the entire lower half of the body may suffer grievous – and not easily-reversed – damage. And as the late Jim Fixx – the world-famous advocate of running, who died quite young of heart failure as he ran – unfortunately proved, even the cardiovascular system may not benefit as much as has been theorized.

Are the results of harsh exercise worth it? Probably not – especially when equal and longer-lasting benefits are available from more gentle and humane programs, such as the one described in the following pages.

Two Types of Exercise

There are essentially two kinds of exercises – commonly (but perhaps a bit incorrectly) called *isometric* and *isotonic* – and several stages or 'levels' of each: gentle . . . moderate . . . and vigorous.

Isometric exercises characteristically pit a number of muscles against an immovable object (such as a heavy weight) or against each other with no appreciable movement for the effort. *Isotonic exercises*, on the other hand, are considered those where the driving effort of muscles moves primarily in one direction or where effort is directed against a movable object. A complete physical exercise program includes both types of exercises with the emphasis being on the isotonic (movement) rather than isometric (static).

Isometric exercises are one important 'leg' of this G-JO INSTITUTE ACUGENICS FITNESS PROGRAM. They build an attractive-looking figure quickly. But because of the kind of process involved, people suffering from any cardiovascular problems (e.g. heart disorders, high blood pressure, etc.) should either avoid this type of exercise or proceed only after their doctor's approval.

About Isotonic Exercises

Gentle isotonic exercises – which form the second leg of The G-JO INSTITUTE ACUGENICS FITNESS PROGRAM – primarily revolve around *stretching* and similar low-movement methods (e.g., 'slow dance', etc.), as well as normal walking, climbing stairs, gardening, or such.

Vigorous isotonic exercises might include longer walks – say, a mile or more at a time – or periods of swimming, bicycling, etc. *Harsh* exercise – running, strenuous calisthenics, and such – plays little part in the following program but may have occasional benefits, especially for those who eat high-protein diets. (High protein diets, which most Westerners eat, cause high levels of stress which, in turn, perpetuate the need for harsh exercise, as noted earlier.)

Running – or other strenuous vigorous movement-type exercises – may provide certain temporary benefits: aggressive energy is burned ... muscular tension may be briefly replaced by 'relaxation' (more typically, *exhaustion*) ... the cardiovascular system is forced to work (but in excess is a powerful abuse!) ... the mind is taken off of self (thus easing depression) ... sweating and breathing functions are stimulated, and a sense of emotional peace, harmony and relaxation temporarily occurs within some individuals (among other benefits).

But anything that running or other harsh exercises can do can be accomplished more easily, gently and enjoyably without much difficulty – and with *much* less effort – using this Acugenics program.

Avoid Harsh Exercise Except Briefly

The traditional Oriental opinion – which is the basis for The G-JO INSTITUTE ACUGENICS FITNESS PROGRAM – holds that while gentle-to-moderate exercise is beneficial, harsh or vigorous exercise may actually be quite harmful and should be avoided unless absolutely necessary. The nature of life is toward rest and quiet rather than movement and chaos; excessive exercise and work are abusive and cause suffering. The only time when harsh exercise is considered at all beneficial is when wrong or excessive foods have been consumed – *eat less, exercise less* (or work less) is a good rule to keep in mind.

Gentle-to-moderate exercise is that which is enough to bring a feeling of invigoration and a *light* sheen of perspiration to the forehead. Moderate-to-heavy exercise is that which brings heavy or profuse perspiration; it has the function of purging and cleansing the system when used 'medicinally'.

It is best to avoid the temptation to undertake a 'body-building' program, especially one which emphasizes weight-lifting and other techniques designed to expand and harden muscles. Not only does such a program require an ever-increasing involvement to maintain one's 'shape', but such programs may actually contribute to arthritis and other degenerative joint and muscular (liver) ailments, not to mention the obesity that plagues a muscular body 'gone to seed'.

Furthermore, as reported in Vol. 12, Issue 7 of *Physician and Sportsmedicine*, two thirds of all fit, young athletes (ages 16 to 33) were found to have blood in the cerebrospinal fluid – the cushion of normally clear fluid that surrounds the brain and spinal cord – soon after weight-lifting. This is an indisputable indication of hemorrhage which occurs from a sudden, massive increase in blood pressure – often as high as 450/380!

While brief periods of harsh or vigorous exercise may temporarily reduce stress and tension, an excess of such exercise quickly tends to *create* stress (in the form of hard or rigid muscles) and may actually eventually contribute to stress-related ailments (e.g. hypertension or high blood pressure, etc.).

Suggested Rules for Vigorous Exercise

If you feel you need vigorous exercise, here are several suggestions that will be beneficial:

* Increase your levels of exercise gradually – don't fall into the trap of 'competing' (against yourself, an arbitrary level, a friend, etc.);
* Change the healthstyle that creates the need for vigorous exercise – reduce stress . . . eat better . . . express love more . . . relax and enjoy . . .
* Do all exercises 'from' the *hara* (also known as *tan tien*, the area approximately two inches below the navel, which is considered to be the center of the human being; *hara* is the 'home' of energy in the body, a reservoir, as well as the meditative point for centering and doing many breathing and relaxation techniques – see below).

An Important Secret of Fitness

Aside from metaphysical reasons for 'focusing' on the *hara* or the lower mid-abdomen during exercising, there is a very practical reason, as well: when the most bulky, 'unsophisticated' muscles (those found in the lower abdomen) are kept supple, flexible and 'in shape', the more sophisticated muscles which radiate outward from there are also invariably in good shape. This 'radiant effect' even travels to the most distant points on the body.

If you had only a single exercise you could do, the best would be one that affects the lower abdomen. The fastest and easiest way to improve and maintain overall health and fitness is to improve the *hara*. When the *hara* is sick, the whole being is sick; when the *hara* is well, complete wellness usually soon follows. (Note: strengthening the *hara* means making it strong, supple and flexible, but not necessarily rigid, hard and well-defined.)

The Primary Function of Movement

Movement (or attempted movement) – that is, exercise – may serve a number of purposes, but ultimately its most important function is to drain stress from the muscles so that *proper relaxation, and thus, proper movement of energy along the meridians*, can occur. The bioenergy meridians run along and within the muscles, so that when muscles are relaxed, the pathways are 'open'; but when muscles are tense and rigid, the meridians are more 'closed'.

Relaxation is the complement of exercise, and a period of rest should always follow *any* kind of exercise routine. Harsh exercise makes resting and relaxing difficult, especially if it is continued to the point where heavy perspiration and harsh or panting breathing occur at that point, the system is loaded with adrenaline – causing the so-called 'runner's high' – which is unsustainably invigorating, and which shortly loads the system with insulin and other 'depressing' chemicals, as a reaction to normalize blood-sugar. Depression (or its companion, *addiction* to the harsh exercise) typically follows. It often becomes a vicious circle. Soon, harsh exercise begins *feeding* stress – just the very thing that mild exercise releases.

Exercise is Only Half a Word

'Exercise' is only half a word: it should be *exercise-and-relaxation*. An ancient – yet complete – Eastern program that incorporates the exercise-and-relaxation theme is *hatha yoga* (or simply 'yoga', to most Westerners).

In hatha yoga, certain bodily postures – called *asanas* – are used to stretch the muscles slightly beyond their normal reach. This releases lactic acid and other muscle-tiring chemicals into the excretory systems of the body, serving the purpose of energy balancing and rejuvenation.

Yoga may be thought of as an integrated method of unifying the body, mind and spirit and emphasizes *flexibility* – not muscular hardness or rigidity – as the means to this end. The purpose of yoga, at least in the tradition that spawned it, is not to glorify the body, but to simply keep it useful and healthy for the purpose of serving its owner well throughout (a hopefully long and happy) life.

Stretching: The Yoga of The West

It is not necessary to learn the *asanas* or postures of yoga to obtain its benefits of fitness and relaxation. This can be accomplished almost as effectively and rather more easily with a regular program of stretching, such as described below.

The yoga postures are not designed to build hard muscles, only to release tension and the muscle-tiring chemicals that stress produces. So stretching also serves the same purpose and function: it allows the muscles to relax and function much better. However, as an aside, some of the best-looking bodies *are* achieved and maintained *only* by a regular program of stretching-type exercise.

Furthermore, stretching takes no lessons nor learning an unfamiliar philosophy – it comes as naturally to us as breathing, blinking or any other unconscious function we do on a regular basis. And like breathing, this unconscious function can be consciously 'overridden' and used deliberately at regular intervals throughout the day to improve our health, fitness and general well-being.

Before You Begin . . .

When seeking to restore health and fitness you must use this guideline: *the more out of shape (ill) you are, the more gentle you must be with yourself in the beginning of any fitness program.*

To plunge into a harsh, demanding fitness program is to invite a normal, protective mechanism – the above-mentioned homeostasis – into action. This is the same mechanism that forces dieters who have undertaken a radical, 'crash' diet to shortly regain as much (and often *more)* weight than the harsh diet lost for them.

Homeostasis is a protective mechanism that helps the mind cope more easily with change and must be considered when planning any long-term fitness and health program. Thus, it is important to begin gently and move gradually toward fitness, if you expect your mind and emotions to cooperate for a meaningful length of time.

As mentioned above, never undertake an exercise program that you cannot realistically commit yourself to for the rest of your life. Don't set ridiculous goals for yourself: becoming fit is only the first, small step – *staying* fit and healthy is much more difficult. In other words, fitness and health is the *way*, not the goal. To paraphrase a wise Oriental pundit: health and fitness are not stations we arrive at – they are means of travelling.

Be gentle, loving and forgiving to yourself: it took your system years to deteriorate, but even with the most gentle program it should only take a matter of several months to restore a high degree of fitness and health. Don't rush – you have the rest of your life.

Section II:
Techniques for Fitness

The G-JO INSTITUTE ACUGENICS FITNESS PROGRAM is an easy-to-use method for restoring/maintaining fitness and health. It is beneficial for people of all ages and in nearly all states of health. But for people who are chronically or seriously ill, this program should be undertaken in a slow and gentle way, adjusted as necessary, for comfort. This program is divided into two parts:

* those techniques which are done on a *daily* basis;
* and those techniques which are done on a *regular-to-occasional* basis.

Part 1: Daily Techniques

The following techniques are done on a daily basis (in many cases being only refinements of activities most of us regularly perform); they are the 'bread-and-butter' of The G-JO INSTITUTE ACUGENICS FITNESS PROGRAM. They include:

* Stretching
* Rest
* Deep breathing techniques
* Gentle isotonic exercise
* Meditative relaxation and visualizing

* 'Energy-balancing' techniques
* Pleasure and play
* RIGHT EATING

How to stretch

Stretching is the key to an effective, 'exercise-less' exercise program. In good health, you need practically nothing more than regular, complete stretching (plus moderate eating) to stay fit, supple and strong. As mentioned earlier, aside from walking, this is the only exercise that most domestic animals receive, yet if they eat moderately, they generally remain strong and agile throughout their lives.

As simple as it is, stretching properly is an art which takes a little practice. The key word to remember is: *slowly*. Stretch as slowly as possible.

As with nearly all the moving or static techniques described in this program, *slow* and *deliberate* stretching (the only kind that is suggested) accomplishes several things. First, it puts less strain on the muscles than sharp, jerky movement, thus avoiding possible injury to the tissues, tendons, ligaments or joints. Also, it actually stimulates the muscles better than fast or chaotic movements (as you will quickly feel).

Long, slow stretching also gives all the muscles – and the connective tissues attached to them – a chance to release the tension and tiring chemicals locked therein. An important Oriental fitness and martial arts program – *t'ai chi ch'uan* – is based on nothing more than a series of slow, specific stretching movements and is practiced by Chinese people of all ages, producing for them remarkable health benefits.

With stretching, the goal is to affect every muscle to a greater or lesser extent, with the main focus being on the muscles of the extremities (hands, feet, etc.), as well as those areas where tension is normally stored (especially the neck, shoulders and lower back). Later, other techniques will be directed to the *hara*, that lower central abdominal area, but stretching is primarily for the more 'sophisticated' and refined muscles.

Proper stretching should cause no pain, only release and sensual pleasure. Next to sexual orgasm and the complete evacuation of the bowels or bladder, a good stretch is one of the most satisfying of all human experiences. Needless to say, it should be enjoyed often – at least several times every day.

Daily stretching techniques

The first stretch of the day should be done in bed. Begin by reaching the arms up toward the ceiling as far as they will go and spread the fingers as widely as they will part. Do this slowly and sensually . . . enjoy the feeling of consciousness returning. Then relax your arms and draw your knees up to your chest and hold this stretch for a few seconds. Again, do it slowly and gently. And to stretch the jaw muscles, add a yawn.

With your knees still drawn up, do a brief massage of your feet and toes. Work them all around using your thumb to massage any sore spots. This is a kind of basic 'micro-acupressure' massage – it has numerous health benefits beyond simply contacting the muscles (this technique is described more completely below).

After doing your deep breathing exercises (see below) and arising, do a *slow* complete body stretch: but begin by briskly shaking the hands loosely from limp wrists long enough until you feel a distinct tingling sensation moving up your arms. This accomplished, stand in a 'tee' position, arms completely outstretched, palms downward. Now *slowly* rotate the palms upward, to face the ceiling and hold for a few moments.

Next, reach both arms as high as you can to the ceiling while bending backward as far as is comfortably possible – again with your fingers widely outstretched (or even better, intertwine the fingers and turn the palms upward toward the ceiling so the fingers are bent somewhat backwards) – and hold for a few seconds. At this point, jut your lower jaw as far forward as possible to stretch the neck muscles. Hold for a few moments, and relax the jaw and return to an upright position. Now gradually bring your arms forward, letting them drop downwards, allowing yourself to slowly hang forward from your waist with your fingers reaching toward the floor (note: as you hang forward, try pulling your abdomen *up and in* to gain additional benefits).

Important: do not force yourself down any further than your body wants to naturally hang from the waist – let gravity gently take you lower and lower as the days and weeks pass. Hang forward this way until it becomes slightly uncomfortable, then gradually straighten up.

You should already be feeling a glowing sense of life and vitality by the time this stretch is finished. Now, put your hands against a wall or chair and take several small steps backwards until your body is angled forward as far as is comfortable from your ankles and calf muscles (this technique is an excellent exercise for helping to prevent nocturnal leg cramps). Hold this for a few seconds, then step forward.

If you have a chair handy, put one foot on that and move the other one back – to do a modified 'split' – then hold for a few seconds, and reverse position. A second alternative is to put one hand against the wall to steady yourself, then draw one knee up to the chest and with the free arm pull it as tightly to the chest as is comfortable. Again, reverse the process, using the other arm and leg, after a few seconds.

Next, slowly turn your neck as far to one side as

possible, allowing your shoulders and upper back to also move to the most comfortable extreme; then reverse directions. And to conclude your stretch allow your head to gradually hang backwards as far as comfortable and move it from one side to the other. Then straighten your head up and open your mouth as widely as you can . . . stick your tongue out as far as possible . . . hold for a few seconds . . . then exhale completely, saying 'haaaa' aloud as you do; now relax your mouth and tongue, then move your jaw slightly from side to side.

While there are many variations of this basic stretching routine, you need nothing more than this to reach and affect virtually all the muscles of the body. As mentioned above, this should be done everyday.

Resting and relaxing

As mentioned earlier the primary reasons for any kind of exercising (including stretching) are threefold: to promote flexibility . . . to keep the energy meridians or pathways operating normally . . . and to allow lactic acid (and other fatigue biochemicals) to drain from the muscles and be excreted, resorbed or converted within the system. A key element necessary for the latter process – fatigue chemical resorption – is to take at least a brief period of rest and relaxation following any exercise, including stretching.

A good rule of thumb is to relax twice as long as the exercise took to complete. It can be as simple as just sitting down for a few minutes – which is wise in the case of stretching – or may even include lying down (this is usually done following a yoga posture).

But there is a much more important period of rest and relaxation that should be made a primary part of any fitness program: the mid-afternoon break (preferably a nap or period of deep meditative relaxation – see below).

This 'siesta' should last for at least 30 minutes . . . and preferably a bit longer.

The body-mind appears to operate best on a diurnal (circadian) rest-cycle basis. That is, two periods of sleep in the 24 hour day. By sleeping (or at least resting) twice a day, it is quite possible to reduce the actual number of hours needed for sleeping by as much as 40%! By sleeping for an hour to 90 minutes during the 'loggy' part of the afternoon, it is quite possible to feel good and rested – assuming one is living a careful healthstyle – with as little as four hours of sleep during the night. And following a twice-a-day sleep program, one finds oneself much more energetic and productive, as an added bonus.

Thus, a minute or two of rest after each period of stretching or exercise plus a second prolonged period of sleep or deep rest is not only important to health and fitness: it also adds enormous pleasure to life.

Deep breathing exercises

Good air is more important than good food – air *is* food: we 'eat' or consume air constantly, while we take solid (or liquid) food only several times a day. There are numerous, well-documented reports of individuals who have lived 40, 50, and even more years without food . . . when they followed certain breathing techniques (e.g., Dr Barbara Moore – an English medical doctor – lived high in the Alps for extensive periods of time on nothing more than air and water).

Obviously, right breathing is more than just getting air into the lungs – even the least healthy of us manages to breathe more or less regularly. Right breathing is a delicate science that requires basic knowledge combined with conscious attention for its proper application.

There are virtually no health disorders which cannot

be relieved, greatly improved or even cured by controlled breathing exercises, according to many traditional Oriental doctor-philosophers. But even the best air is of little value if not 'consumed' properly; on the other hand, the negative effects of polluted air are greatly diminished with the following techniques.

The science and technique of right breathing

Right breathing begins with the nostrils – not the mouth. While it is possible, of course, to bring air into the lungs by way of the mouth, there are certain vital functions which are performed by nasal breathing:

* Membranes of the sinuses are stimulated, which in turn has a stimulating effect on the area of the brain that is responsible for psychic and creative activity;
* Air is pre-warmed – or cooled – to closely duplicate the body's temperature before reaching the lungs;
* The pituitary gland – and, secondarily, the pineal gland – are also stimulated as breath passes up the nostrils, etc., which regulates and improves vital endocrine functions.

(Note: we seldom breathe equally with both nostrils at the same time; instead, the pattern is a more-or-less alternating cycle, first through the right nostril for several hours, then more through the left, depending on the time of day, state of emotions, etc. Breathing through the *right* nostril has a cooling effect; through the *left* nostril, a warming effect. Often you will find that one nostril or the other 'breathes more easily'; if it is the right nostril, you probably tend to have cold feet; if it is the left, you probably tend to be warm.)

A good method for deep breathing

There are a number of deep breathing exercises, ranging from simple to complex (and each has a different effect on the body-mind); but most of these methods stress breathing 'from' the lower abdomen (the *hara*) or even 'deeper' (e.g., 'from' the heels). What this means is to imagine (and actually 'feel') breath being drawn as deeply as the navel (or the heels or toes) – rather than just to the lungs – when you inhale. This tends to activate the abdominal muscles (which are essential muscles for properly operating the breathing mechanisms of the upper chest). It also keeps attention focused on the *hara*.

A second important technique – one which you probably don't do unless you've had special training – is to breathe *with the tip of your tongue curled back into the roof (palate) of your mouth*. This is one of the most important Oriental health techniques to reach the West; it is simple to do and – after a short time – becomes an automatic way of breathing. Some of its many benefits are:

* aiding digestion . . .
* easing thirst . . .
* helping to keep one emotionally centered . . .
* helping stimulate the heart (the tongue is 'connected' to the heart, in traditional Oriental philosophy), as well as the stomach, to aid digestion.

The purpose of deep breathing is to '*balance energy*'. Energy is *activated* by *inhalation*. And energy is *relaxed* by *exhalation*. Furthermore, energy is 'raised' through short, fast breaths and is calmed through long, slow breaths. Energy is *controlled* or 'balanced' by *retaining* (holding) the breath. What this means is that it is difficult to be relaxed when breathing quickly and hard to be tense when breathing slowly: the slower we breathe and the longer we pause between breaths, the more relaxed we become.

The following exercises are generally done for ten complete breathing cycles twice a day, and may be repeated more frequently, if desired. Since 'relearning' to breathe takes sustained, conscious effort, in the beginning you must set aside at least several minutes twice a day just for breathing. Later, you will find yourself unconsciously breathing much more deeply and slowly . . . even with the tip of your tongue tucked snugly into the roof of your mouth.

When you deep-breathe, breathe. Do nothing else (except, perhaps, some gentle exercise). Begin your breathing exercise with empty lungs; then fill them according to the directions below. When you exhale, drain yourself as completely as possible (draining not only your lungs but your stress and tension, as well).

The one-two-one-two cycle

The 'basic' Acugenics deep breathing exercise is called 'the one-two-one-two cycle': here, you fill your lungs slowly and deeply to the count of four, five, six or even longer (this is the 'one' part of the cycle); then hold your breath for *twice* that number (e.g. eight, ten, twelve, etc.); then exhale to the same count that you inhaled, making sure to drain the lungs as completely as possible; and retain a state of 'no-breath' for the same, long count as when you held your breath at the 'top' of the cycle.

A good beginning cycle is a four-count inhale, an eight-count retention, a four-count exhale and an eight-count no-breath retention. If this is too uncomfortable, reduce it to a three-six-three-six cycle; or if it feels just a bit rushed, increase it to a five-ten-five-ten cycle, and build your tolerances gradually.

The 'weak lungs' variation

A useful variation of the basic deep breathing cycle, for a person with weak lungs, is to *inhale* long breaths, deeply and slowly through the nostrils as normal . . . then retain. But *exhale* through tightly-pursed lips (as if blowing through a narrow straw or whistle) as hard as is comfortably possible for the same count of time that the breath is held or the no-breath state is retained. This would then be a 'one-two-*two*-two' cycle. This variation is particularly useful for smokers and others who have inhaled abusive substances for long periods of time.

A further variation of that same, pursed-lips exhale is to blow at the leaves of a plant or a piece of paper, increasing the distance just enough to keep the 'target' moving throughout the exhaling.

The Institute of Breathing variations

There are two deep breathing exercises taught by the Institute of Breathing (England), which are similar to the above.

Sit in a chair, hands on thighs, with the back straight . . . inhale to the count of seven . . . pause one second . . . exhale deeply . . . pause another second . . . and repeat this again (up to seven times per session).

Or lie on your back, knees drawn partially up and slightly apart . . . inhale deeply, allowing the abdomen to rise and fill up like a balloon, first . . . then purse the lips, exhaling slowly but forcefully until the diaphram is pushed into the chest . . . then puff the last bit of air out . . . and repeat.

How to test your lungs

The goal of any deep breathing exercise is to increase the capacity of the lungs: when lung capacity is increased, we automatically breathe more deeply and completely. To know just how much you need to use a breathing development program, there are two good tests to measure the fitness of your lungs.

First, take a deep breath and hold it: now with a cloth tape measure, measure the distance around your chest and back at the level of the nipples . . . then exhale as much air as possible and measure your chest again at the same level. The difference between the two measurements should be at least 2½ inches for a woman and 3½ inches for a man; the larger the difference, the greater the capacity of your lungs.

Another test is to take a deep breath and simply hold it as long as you can: the average time for most people is about 55 seconds. Now exhale as deeply as you can and don't breathe again until you have to. The average length of time for holding out is about 15 seconds. (Note: the pulse rate is another basic indicator of the state of one's fitness. In an adult male, the 'resting' – or 'first-thing-in-the-morning' – pulse rate should be between 60 and 70 beats per minute; in an adult female, from 65 to 75 beats per minute. Pulse rate is generally faster in a child – up to 140 beats per minute for newborn infants – but generally slower than normal in very healthy adults.)

When to do deep breathing exercises

The best time to do your first deep breathing exercises is in the morning, either while you are still in bed or immediately upon arising (just after your stretching exercises is a perfect time). This will help the waking-up process proceed smoothly and provide you with plenty of energy for the rest of the morning.

At least one more cycle of deep breathing should be done during (or just after) the mid-afternoon 'doldrums', especially if you are not able to take a rest or siesta during that time. If you *can* rest, do your second cycle afterwards.

But avoid any deep breathing exercises within an hour or two before going to bed – unless they are relaxing-type breaths (slow, deep exhales) – or you may not be able to fall quickly asleep due to feeling 'too much energy'.

About daily isotonic exercising

As mentioned earlier, exercising essentially means 'movement'. While there are a number of specific exercises suggested for The G-JO INSTITUTE ACUGENICS FITNESS PROGRAM (see below), these are primarily of the *isometric* form and are not suggested for daily use (at least after the first several weeks of beginning this program).

If you are leading a normal life – which means walking at least several hundred steps a day, perhaps climbing a flight or two of steps regularly or doing a reasonable amount of housework or gardening – you are probably getting enough movement-type exercise . . . especially if you combine it with the stretching techniques and energy-balancing exercises incorporated in the program.

Furthermore, there are ways of additionally increasing the amount of exercise you normally get without altering your daily patterns substantially. First, you can walk up several sets of steps when you might ordinarily take an elevator or escalator. Or you might choose to walk to the next bus stop or arrange to have someone pick you up an extra block away from your normal meeting spot. Perhaps it could mean carrying a report to someone yourself, rather than sending a secretary to do it . . . the opportunities are limitless, with just a little bit of thought.

How much exercising to do

The goal is to walk a minimum of three or four hundred steps a day. Walking is one of the most complete movement-type exercises there is, and should be an integral part of any health program. Climbing steps adds additional movement of certain muscles and has many benefits for the cardiovascular system.

To gain even more benefit from walking, imagine a fishing line tied from your belt buckle (or coming out from your navel to a 'winch' or a 'reel' at your destination. Then while walking, imagine someone at your destination 'reeling you in' (like a fish) as you walk. The benefits? An immediate improvement in posture . . . a surprising increase in speed (great if you're a runner!) . . . and you'll use less energy to walk farther or faster.

Incidentally, you can also improve posture by picturing yourself with a long pony-tail that is being pulled up from the top of your head, to an imaginary point directly above you in the sky.

Still another technique – one that combines both relaxation and movement – is *rocking in a rocking chair.* Gentle though it may be, pushing a rocking chair for an hour or so provides numerous benefits for the entire lower half of the body as well as the cardiovascular system, etc. . . . and it may be done while watching TV, reading or even doing many kinds of paperwork. Thus, daily exercising need not be boring, fatiguing nor require anything other than a slight variation of perhaps your normal patterns.

The mind's role in exercise

The mind plays an active role in gaining the most benefits from small amounts of gentle exercise. By paying attention to what you are doing and 'focusing' on (mentally directing energy to) the general bodily area you wish to exercise, your mind will receive – and follow – your orders to improve that area.

As mentioned earlier, the *hara* – or center – of the body, located about two inches below the navel, should be the central focus point for all exercising. This means, when walking, breathing, or doing any specific exercise, try to imagine yourself incorporating these activities 'to' or 'from' that key area below your navel (such as the deep breathing or 'fishing reel' techniques described above). Another technique (described below) utilizes the mind's powerful 'visualizing' capabilities.

This technique – called 'mind-picturing' – can actually help you 'sculpt' the body you want . . . almost without effort. And it really works!

Combine exercises for more benefits

You can gain extra benefits by consciously doing additional deep breathing exercises for the full amount of time that you are exercising. Not only is this an easy way to do these exercises, but it gives you the opportunity to add several more 'breathing sessions' to your daily routine.

Even the simple act of chewing – when done thoughtfully – becomes an important part of daily exercise. By chewing a minimum of 30 times per bite you provide benefits not only to the jaw, but (and much more important) to the *liver* and ultimately to the entire muscular system (which the liver is said to control, according to Oriental doctor-philosophers). Proper chewing also has the added benefit of improving one's sex life (due to the effect on the liver – a main 'control' organ also for sexual drive and vigor).

Meditative relaxation

Applied, *deep* relaxation – *meditative* relaxation – combines deep rest and a special visualizing technique to utilize this state of relaxation to improve fitness and health. In the Orient it is said that mental therapies are superior to physical therapies . . . that sometimes simply mentally picturing that which you want (in this case, a more fit and healthy body) is enough to achieve your goals – as long as you do it diligently, regularly and with as much concentration as possible.

As you perfect this method, you should incorporate it into your daily routine *twice* a day. Ideally, it is best to use that period of time just between waking and sleeping – or between sleeping and waking – to both relax and, more important, mentally visualize the state of mind and body you desire. But this technique can actually be done *any* time of the day or night with good results.

How to unlock the mind's awesome power

'Visualizing' or 'mind-picturing' means simply *making*, *holding* and *expanding* a somewhat distorted and vivid mental 'picture' of yourself as you want to become . . . or to stay (see below).

This technique serves several purposes. First, it creates a 'mind photograph' that your enormous subconscious powers can use as a model (and these will indeed eventually 'sculpt' your body to rather fit your mind's specifications, because *form eventually follows thought* – this is one of the primary and most valid metaphysical laws). Visualization also reinforces the mental commitment to improve fitness and health.

Meditative relaxation is nothing more than the act of stopping, sitting or lying down and turning inward. To do it properly, first get in a comfortable position and tightly clench *all* your muscles at the same time and hold for a few seconds. Then relax the muscles and begin counting from one to ten. With each number, 'will' a specific part of your body to release tension and become completely relaxed (e.g., at the count of one, relax your feet . . . on two, your lower legs . . . on three, your knees and upper legs or thighs, etc.). When you reach ten, you should be quite relaxed and ready to 'visualize' the message to your mind. (Note: certain G-Jo acupressure points illustrated and described in Section III may also be used to deepen relaxation, due to their effects on various muscles. These are called 'Meditative Relaxation' points and, if used, should be first triggered for a few seconds each before beginning the relaxation process.)

Making a vivid 'mind-picture'

The key to good visualization, once you are deeply relaxed, is to paint a vivid (if rather distorted) mind-picture of that body shape or state of health and fitness which you desire for yourself. For instance, if you wish to be lean, trim and lithe, see yourself as not only lean and limber, but make yourself even absurdly skinny, in your mind, and able to do amazing feats of gymnastics. See yourself actually *doing* these remarkable feats – feats that only a circus acrobat or comic book hero can perform.

Let yourself 'feel' in your mind, to the best of your ability, your acts of gymnastics and the wonderful sensation it would be to have exactly the kind of body and ability which you picture in your mind's eye. Let the picture unfold in slow-motion, feeling as completely as possible the effortless freedom and power your mind gives you. You are only limited – or, better, *unlimited* – by your imagination.

Understand this: the part of the mind we need to use to sustain our drive toward health and fitness (namely, the subconscious) is best reached by vivid emotionalism, not logic. Thus, don't worry if your mind-picture doesn't 'make sense' – your subconscious will understand and respond accordingly . . . if you 'drive' this desire deep into your subconscious by repeating your 'thought-movie' often enough.

With nearly any ailment (or loss of fitness) there are corresponding, unnatural muscle 'sets' or arrangements (tension), which can cause/perpetuate symptoms, dysfunction or discomfort. Conversely, by 'willing' the tension to 'depart' we can control, relieve and erase many of the symptoms that we suffer . . . as well as increasing our fitness and health. Using meditative relaxation techniques is one of the most crucial steps in the ACUGENICS FITNESS PROGRAM – make sure you use them often!

Energy-balancing techniques

Almost as important as the mental and visualizing techniques are the uniquely Oriental energy-balancing methods as practiced by Taoists – those who follow the principles of the Chinese philosopher, Lao Tsu, as described in his classic, the *Tao Te Ching* – for countless centuries. There are many of these easy-to-do 'exercises' – perhaps hundreds of them!

But by knowing – and applying – even just the few described below, you will receive many important benefits. The primary purpose of these methods is *life extension*. That is, to extend a life that would normally be shortened by abusive practices, ignorance or foolish ways of living to a life that lasts its normal measure (which, according to Taoists, is at least one hundred years). Several of these practices have already been described – shaking the hands loosely from the wrists until energy is felt to be 'flowing' – and jutting the jaw as far forward as possible while the neck is stretched (which stimulates the entire endocrine system). But several other methods should also be incorporated into your daily practices (perhaps at the same time you do your stretching).

The first one is called *scalp-tapping*. Here, you simply tap all around your scalp using the tips of the fingers in a drumming kind of a motion. The process should be slightly painful (which stimulates the scalp acupuncture system) but need only last for a few moments.

The next technique could be called the 'nose-wobble'. Here, you grasp and tweak and wobble the nose briskly until a slight numbness occurs thereupon. This may be easily done in the shower or while washing the face and provides the benefit of stimulating the acupuncture system of the nose.

A third, easy technique is to tap the fingertips briskly on the face, paying special attention to the area around the mouth. Here, you should tap deeply enough to feel stimulation in the teeth and gums – all of which are somehow connected to specific, inner organs and glands. By tapping these areas briskly, you are actually having an effect on those underlying or connected organs and glands. (Note: if you have long fingernails, use your knuckles as if you were knocking on a door to stimulate these areas.)

One of the most powerful acupuncture systems is found in the *ears*. There are more than two hundred tiny acupuncture points located in either ear and a complete system of healing – based on nothing more than 'triggering' these points with a toothpick, a needle or other tool – has a long history of success in the Orient.

But you can give yourself a simple 'tune-up' of this system by simply pulling and yanking the top, lobe and back of either ear in a brisk but gentle manner. Finish this technique by 'tracing' with the fingertip or -nail around all the ridges and crevasses found within the ear.

The last of these simple energy-balancing methods is to *deeply squeeze and pinch* the tips of each finger and toe (just behind and beside the nail). Invariably, you will find several of these fingers or toe tips to be rather tender – pay the most attention to these as you massage. Each finger and toe is connected to an inner organ or gland, just as are various other appendages throughout the body. By stimulating the tips of the fingers and toes we are, again, helping to restore balance and harmony to each inner organ or gland.

While the entire series of energy-balancing techniques takes less than 2 or 3 minutes to perform, the effects last for many hours afterwards. In fact, regularly performing these energy-balancing methods has many long-term benefits, too. Ailments – even long-standing chronic disorders – are often dramatically relieved, when these methods are incorporated into our daily practices for at least several months. In any event, they are safe . . . easy to perform . . . and can produce only good results – especially when they become a regular part of your healthstyle.

Pleasure and play

Too often we approach the chore of gaining/maintaining fitness with the same seriousness as we would in pursuing a materialistic goal. However, health and fitness are the way, the path, and not simply an end-point (although human nature is such as to put it in those simple terms). While dedication and discipline are vital for a life-long successful fitness program, without a deep sense of pleasure and play, it becomes a meaningless gesture. Fitness for its own sake is an empty state of being and body-worship.

Fitness and health are simply states of *freedom from suffering* which allow a person, if he so chooses, to more diligently pursue the ultimate purpose of his life (which, in the traditional Oriental point of view, is to 'achieve' the state *spiritual enlightenment*). An integral part of this sense of spiritual peace is *contentment*, which invariably includes frequent doses of pleasure and play.

This may be as simple as giving yourself permission to enjoy at least one pleasurable activity per day (which you might have denied yourself before), or it may mean even radically changing your life to make room for your beautiful, growing sense of self-confidence. But without adding more pleasure and play to your life, the whole point of fitness and health is lost.

Right eating for health and fitness

As described earlier, right eating is by far the most important key to total body-mind health and fitness. As mentioned, the best diet – that is, the one which is least taxing to our electro-chemical system – is *vegetarian*, based on whole grains (especially whole or brown rice).

But if you are moving toward the meatless way of eating, especially if you are living a 'normal' Western lifestyle (meaning one relatively high in stress), it is vital to learn proper *food combining techniques*. Stress primarily affects (and is affected *by*) the state of our kidneys and adrenals. These, in turn, are most dramatically affected by the amount and type of proteins (as well as the *salt*) we consume.

Too much – especially too much *animal-based* –

protein causes stress. But an insufficient protein intake will eventually cause 'burn-out' (low energy, malnutrition, etc.). This is especially true if we try to continue a high-stress lifestyle as our diet becomes 'low stress'. So proper food combining is essential for *beginning* vegetarians to insure enough usable protein to sustain a healthful life (later, however, as the healthstyle adjusts itself, the need for protein is greatly reduced).

Proper food combining means mixing whole grains, legumes, dairy products or other common, non-slaughtered foods to form complete protein.

The key to right eating is, of course, *moderation.* While it is best to eat regionally and seasonally (that is, selecting fresh food grown locally), even 'unhealthy' foods and substances may generally be safely taken in moderation . . . assuming no 'hidden' allergy to them exists.

If you live a 'normal' life – meaning a 9-to-5 job, regular activities and a not-too-careful diet – it is best to eat five or six *small* meals (vs. two or three *larger* ones) daily. It is best to take not more than three kinds of foods per meal; and make the biggest meals earlier in the day, with the smaller meals coming later. There are numerous possible rules and suggestions for healthful eating, but the most important one to remember is simple: *eat moderately*.

As mentioned earlier, suggested healthful, vegetarian recipes whose focus is on complete protein and/or quick energy will be found in Section IV of this manual.

Part 2: Regular and Occasional Fitness Techniques

Unlike the above daily techniques – which are mainly extensions of natural processes we do each day – the following techniques require a break from normal activities and need a period of time (daily in the beginning, then at least every several days, after health and fitness have been restored) for them to be performed.

These techniques – which are the basis for THE ACUGENICS FITNESS PROGRAM – fall into three, main categories:

* Isometric exercises;
* Moderate isotonic exercises;
* Self-massage (including G-Jo acupressure).

Isometric exercises

These are, as described earlier, static (motionless) exercises which pit one muscle or group of muscles against another, the net result being effort without movement. There are certain rules that are absolutely essential to follow, not only for these exercises to be effective, but also to avoid potential injury:

* Do each of the following exercises slowly and gently, gradually increasing pressure over the 'holding' period . . . don't jerk muscles against – or slam them at – each other;
* Do these exercises for only a few seconds at a time (10 seconds *maximum* . . . and that, only after several weeks of conditioning);
* Do these exercises on the *exhale* cycle of breathing, only;
* Repeat these exercises a *maximum* of several times daily (though once a day is generally enough);
* Do these exercises only hard enough to feel the tension and exertion, not so hard that you sense injury done to yourself;
* *Avoid* isometric exercises if you suffer from *any*

cardiovascular disorders (high blood pressure, heart disease, history of stroke, etc.), unless approved by your doctor.

There are ten isometric exercises in this program. They take less than a minute to do completely and may be done in conjunction with other activities (e.g., while watching TV, in a movie – even while stopped at a stop light in your car . . .). They need not disrupt your day in any way. These exercises should be memorized, using short names to describe their actions (after you memorize these names and exercises, you need not refer to this manual):

'LIFTING KNEES' – while seated, place the palms of your hands against your knees and, while pressing down against the knees, attempt to lift your knees to your chest. To increase its effectiveness even further, before trying to lift the knees, raise the heels so you are sitting 'on tip-toes'. Use this exercise *cautiously* . . . if abused, it may cause temporary constipation, hemorrhoidal irritation (if you have hemorrhoids), other ano-genital disorders or create strain on the lower back and abdomen; but in moderation it will strengthen these areas. Of all the isometric exercises, this is the most important since it directly strengthens the *hara*;

'PUSHING HANDS, PULLING HANDS' – while seated, place the palms of your hands against each other at chest-level so the hands are in the 'praying' position, fingers pointing upwards, and press tightly together; then gently release, and hook the fingers of one hand against the fingers of the other and attempt to pull them apart. Finally, reverse the positions of the hands (so the upper hand now becomes the lower and vice-versa), and again attempt to 'unhook' the fingers by pulling against each other (this exercise reaches many of the muscles of the neck, upper torso, shoulders, arms, and hands);

'PUSH DOWN/LIFT UP' – with the top hand's palm facing the floor, place the other palm against it and lift while resisting and pushing downward with the upper; then reverse hands and perform the same exercise (this will strengthen and firm the muscles of the arms and shoulders as well as those of the wrist and hands). Finally, do the same process with either hand, but with the palm of the *lower* hand also facing the floor;

'PUSH LEGS' – while seated with your legs slightly spread apart and feet flat on the floor, press your palms against the outside of your legs near the knees; then try pushing your knees together with your hands while resisting with the legs and attempting to spread them open (this exercises the muscles of the thighs, abdomen, arms, chest and shoulders);

'PULL LEGS' – still seated with your legs slightly spread and feet flat against the floor, hook your fingers on the inside of the legs near the knees; then attempt to pull the legs wider open while resisting and pulling them ever more tightly closed (this exercise affects muscles of the thighs, arms, neck, hips, buttocks and, of course, the fingers);

'HOLD HEAD' – interlock the fingers at the back of the head and pull forward while pushing back with the head and neck (this affects muscles of the arms, neck, shoulders and scalp primarily, as well as other muscles in the trunk of the body, secondarily – *use this exercise cautiously*!);

'PRESS HEAD' – press the palm of the right hand

against the right side of the head, then press each against the other; then duplicate the exercise on the left side: finally, press both palms against the forehead and push that against the hands, which are resisting and pushing against the forehead (this exercises other muscles of the neck, face, arms, shoulders and upper back – as above, *use cautiously*);

'*SIT UP*' – lying on the back, pull the knees up (but keep the feet flat on the floor); then clasp hands behind the neck and attempt to sit up; hold the 'sitting up' position for as long as possible;

'ABDOMINAL LIFT' – standing with your feet about shoulder-width apart, bend your knees slightly and lean forward from the waist far enough to place the palms of your hands on your thighs just above the kneecaps. Force all the air from your lungs, placing the weight of your body on your arms, suck your abdomen in and upwards, keeping the air out of the lungs; pull the navel up towards the spine as far as you can, creating a deep hollow in the abdominal area. Remember – this should be done with all your breath exhaled and holding the no-breath state. In normal health, up to ten of these a day may be performed. (Note: this technique should be avoided if you suffer from high blood pressure, ulcers, heart disorders or during the menstrual period or pregnancy.)

'P-C SQUEEZE AND CLENCH' – tightly squeeze the sphincter muscles of the rectum and urinary outlet (the 'p-c' or pubococcygeal muscles) as tightly as possible and hold for a few seconds; while holding these muscles clenched, also squeeze and clench the muscles of the buttocks together. (Beyond affecting the muscles of the hips and buttocks, this is the second most important exercise of the series and is a very effective method for improving the flow of energy, especially to the sexual organs, the prostate gland in males and for over-all excretion control, etc.) This technique may easily be combined with the above-mentioned 'Abdominal Lift'.

There are numerous variations of these isometric exercises that you may discover on your own and add to your routine as you desire. However, always remember to incorporate at least these basic ten techniques for a complete muscle work-out.

Moderate isotonic (movement) exercises

While there are numerous isotonic – that is, classical movement-type – exercises, there are two in particular (and a third, optional technique) that serve many functions yet may be done by people of all ages quite easily and enjoyably. They are called:

* 'Slow dance';
* 'Swinging arms'

and the third, optional technique (for stronger people) is:

* 'Sit-backs' (or even better, 'sit-ups').

'SLOW DANCE' – this is a Westernized version of the famous Chinese *t'ai chi ch'uan* exercises, mentioned earlier. Essentially, this is nothing more (nor less) than a free-form modern dance routine – done as slowly as possible (to about the same beat or rhythm as religious or Gregorian chants – in other words, nearly as slow as is practical to maintain balance without strain).

Here, the goal is a combination of gentle movement plus stretching: reach high . . . pirouette and stretch your legs . . . bend gently in a slow and graceful manner

. . . move freely, *but slowly* – preferably outdoors, barefoot in the sunlight and dressed in loose, comfortable cotton clothing. For added benefits, keep your spine and neck as straight as possible throughout your session.

While it might seem more rewarding to do harsh, fast jazz- or aerobic-type exercises, the purpose of slow dance is much different than the other, calisthenic-type dance routines. With slow dance, balancing and harmonizing energy – the ultimate effect of most movement (whether done consciously as exercise or not) – is the primary goal. Speed works not for – but against – harmonious flow of vital energy within the system.

This routine should be done until you feel a light sheen of perspiration form across the brow or upper shoulders – about 5 or 6 minutes maximum, and even less for most beginners. The energy-balancing benefits of a slow-dance routine will last for at least several hours, perhaps longer, depending on your subsequent activities and emotions.

While 'slow dance' sounds almost too easy to do, it is actually surprisingly complex – especially if done with full upward and outward stretching – and should only be done to the point just before discomfort arises. The greater the range of movement and the slower the movement, the broader the benefits. Be expressive and creative: imagine yourself as a blade of grass or a dancing fire . . . as you move, focus on your *hara* and think of nothing other than the movement itself (this is also a good time to do your deep breathing exercises, although you should also spend some quiet time breathing for full effectiveness).

Keep in mind 'the Rule of the Four S's': do all movement exercise *slowly* . . . go only *slightly* beyond what is comfortable when exercising (do only *slightly* taxing techniques) . . . do any exercising for only *short* periods of time . . . do only *simple* movements – keep all exercise programs simple and easy to do. In other words: *S*low; *S*ensual; *S*hort; and *S*imple.

'SWINGING ARMS' – while standing with feet at about shoulder width, let the arms hang loosely with the *palms facing forward*; now begin swinging them gently forward and upward to about shoulder height, then swing back as far as they naturally want to go *without forcing them* (make sure to keep the palms facing forward at all times). Repeat this swinging until you feel the effort in the neck, shoulders and sense the energy flowing throughout your arms (40-50 arm swings for most people). This benefits the entire upper body, lymph system and helps prevent many serious diseases, according to its Chinese practitioners. This is a good technique to use before any other, since it is a good 'warm-up' method.

'SIT-BACKS' – this optional technique greatly benefits the lower abdomen with relatively little effort. While seated on the floor with legs stretched in front of you (and possibly with your feet hooked beneath a heavy chair or dresser), and with the arms outstretched or, better, locked behind the neck, *slowly* ease yourself back to a lying down position. Then sit back up. If necessary, help yourself return to the sitting position with your hands, then repeat the process. Gradually build yourself to the point of slowly 'sitting back' only about $\frac{3}{4}$ of the way down and holding that position for a few moments. This makes it both an isotonic *and* an isometric technique. Hold – and repeat – only as long as it causes no undue strain. There are many variations of sit-backs or sit-ups, but this is one of the best. However, it takes some strength and may not be well-suited for all individuals immediately – use common sense!

Other good exercises

There are numerous other isotonic exercises that are both gentle and effective in improving and maintaining fitness. Some of them are:

* Hand circles – with arms outstretched to either side (like a 'Tee'), let the hands hang loosely from the wrists and make small, complete and rapid clockwise circles; then repeat in the opposite direction;
* Neck stretch – stretch your neck up slowly and gently, then turn your head as far as you can from side to side in the process (this should be repeated only a few times);
* 'Picking grapes' – reach as high as you can, standing on tip-toes – stretching upward first with one arm, then the other, reaching and grasping as if you were trying to pick a piece of fruit just beyond your reach.

There are many other easy exercises which may be added, now and then, for fun or variety. However, a bit of walking, stretching, isometric exercises, slow dance and energy-balancing methods are all that most people need to stay fit and healthy . . . especially when other parts of their 'healthstyle' are in order.

In all, these exercises should take no more than 20 minutes, and may be occasionally abbreviated to take less than 5. Even so, they will give you a good workout.

Self-massage techniques

Almost everyone enjoys touching and being touched. This is a natural response that we are born with, and one that may bring numerous therapeutic benefits as well as sensual pleasures. There are several touching techniques which have an important place in THE G-JO INSTITUTE ACUGENICS FITNESS PROGRAM.

As described earlier there are complete acupuncture (healing) systems found in many areas of the body. Two of the most easily manipulated are found on either hand and foot. 'Triggering' these systems into action is a simple process: all we need to do is *deeply* massage the tops, bottoms and sides of the hands and feet, paying particular attention, as mentioned, to the tips of each finger and toe (that is, just behind and to either side of the nail).

Hand and foot massage should be done at least every several days, but not necessarily daily. Its benefits are subtle, but far-reaching. Rather than controlling vital energy flow by movement and other above-described techniques, when we do hand or foot massage we are directly connecting (by so-called 'reflexes') with each of the vital organs and glands.

As an aside, not only is this a good self-massage method, but it is a pleasant and sensual way to relate to a mate, a family member or a special friend.

Other self-massage techniques

There are also, as detailed in the section on 'energy-balancing' methods, complete acupuncture systems on the nose, the ears, the scalp, face and spine (not to mention the arms, abdomen and thighs, etc.). Each of these may be occasionally and briskly massaged with good benefit.

A *scalp massage* is one of the most relaxing and enjoyable pleasures that can occur in the human body. Not only will this have health benefits on the inner organs (especially when you stimulate any tender points you may feel on your scalp), but it also helps promote a head of healthy hair as well as relieving stress (the scalp is a key 'stash' area for carrying tension). Fifteen or twenty seconds of fingertip stimulation is often enough to provide these benefits.

Like other forms of self-massage, this technique should be performed every several days without fail. Again, its goal and purpose is to 'unblock' key acupuncture points in that region to allow unhindered energy flow. It may easily be done while shampooing the hair, but feels better if a special partner does it for you.

Spinal massage is another profoundly-effective healing and health maintenance technique. Here, the most tender spots along either side of the spine – ranging from the upper neck to the buttocks – are deeply triggered for only a moment or two by your partner.

Have your partner probe with his/her thumb tips down either side of your spine until a tender point is found then have your partner massage the spot as deeply as can be tolerated, for several seconds. Finally, continue working downwards. This is a very effective form of acupuncture without needles (or 'acupressure', the subject of the next section of this program and also of many of this author's other publications). As with the above, this technique should also be done every few days and takes only a short time to do. As an aside, this same method can also be very beneficial for your dog or cat. Simply massage any 'ouch points' (or pet 'hot spots') along either side of the spine for a few seconds every few days.

G-Jo acupressure techniques

G-JO ACUPRESSURE is a kind of acupuncture – but without the needles. Whenever the body suffers an illness or injury, tenderness in the body's 'acupressure points' that control or heal the ailment also spontaneously occurs. G-Jo is performed by triggering and massaging these tiny, pressure-sensitive spots located just beneath the skin. Nearly always, the most sensitive of these acupressure points are the ones which are most effective in bringing relief. And, since it is only the body which heals itself, these same techniques often also stimulate the body's own self-healing mechanisms. Acupressure is the most powerful, effective and fastest-acting 'self-health' technique known to man.

To use acupressure for yourself, first look at the appropriate illustrations which accompany this manual. Then – with the tip of the thumb, the bent knuckle of the pointer finger or the eraser tip of a pencil – press the corresponding area on your own body until you feel a sharp or far-reaching twinge of sensitivity. It should feel like a toothache or a pinched nerve. Any particularly tender or sensitive points should be circled on the chart(s) for future reference. After the first session, trigger only those points which are the most sensitive and/or produce the strongest acupressure reactions.

Once the point is located, it is then massaged using goading, moderate-to-deep pressure until an 'acupressure reaction' occurs. This is usually a feeling of warmth, a flush of clamminess, perspiration or a similar response. This reaction usually occurs sometime within the first 30 seconds of stimulating the acupressure point. As soon as this reaction occurs, stop triggering the point; then find – and trigger – the identical point on the opposite side of the body (if applicable). If no reaction occurs, it usually means you are not quite on the acupressure point or that this point is not useful in bringing relief or stimulating self-healing.

Trigger these points symptomatically – that is, only when the symptoms arise – and re-trigger the 'best' (most tender, responsive) points if or when the symptom returns. Generally, G-Jo acupressure should usually not be needed more than four or five times daily. Continue using acupressure until the sensitivity at the points is reduced.

If acupressure produces a particularly strong reaction – such as nausea, faintness or light-headedness – use less pressure for a shorter period of time. Stop if you must, but remember: the points that produce the strongest reactions are usually the best to bring relief and promote self-healing.

However, acupressure should generally be avoided by: *pregnant women* (esp. beyond the third month of pregnancy); *chronic heart patients* (esp. those fitted with pacemaker or similar energy-regulating devices); and *people who take regular or daily medication* (esp. for serious problems, such as cancer or diabetes). Also, you should generally wait about four hours after taking any drugs, medications, alcohol or other intoxicants before applying acupressure.

Furthermore, you should wait about half an hour after eating a hot meal, doing strenuous exercises, or performing heavy labor before applying acupressure. Avoid any acupressure points that fall beneath scars, moles, warts, varicose veins, etc. If your symptoms persist, see your doctor. For more acupressure information, see THE NATURAL HEALER'S ACUPRESSURE HANDBOOK (VOLUMES I and II), also by Michael Blate – from this publisher.

(Note: to trigger acupressure points located in the ear, use a blunt tooth-pick, a match stick or similar tools, and press gently in the approximate area until a deeply-sensitive spot is felt. Then stimulate the point in a gently, rocking or back-and-forth manner. Follow the same guidelines as described above.)

Acupressure eye exercises

A particularly useful acupressure technique – one performed twice daily by most schoolchildren in China – is highly beneficial for the eyes.

Here, you gently but briskly stimulate a series of acupressure points on the hands and face, especially surrounding the eyes (see illustration in Section III). This series of six exercises is done to an eight-count; that is, each point is triggered eight times in a moderate, goading fingertip massage. If done properly, this powerful exercise takes only seconds to perform. But it has worthwhile benefits for improving and maintaining eyesight. (Note: if you wear glasses or contacts and notice headaches or nausea within a few weeks after beginning this program, it may mean your eyes are becoming strong enough to change prescription or even eliminate your glasses, altogether.)

Occasional (medicinal) techniques

Occasionally, we may want to do certain techniques to restore ourselves, especially if we have been neglectful of our healthstyle. Or sometimes they simply feel good to do. While there may be numerous 'occasional' or medicinal health techniques that serve as well, here are two in particular to consider:

* Vigorous exercise;
* Fasting.

* VIGOROUS EXERCISE – as the name implies, this would include nearly any brisk, rapid movement-type activity that brings about profuse perspiration, 'adrenaline rush' or extreme invigoration and other 'symptoms' of cardiovascular, muscular and respiratory exertion.

These are often in the form of sports or recreational

activities. As with most other forms of human activity, *moderation* is the key to vigorous exercise. It is probably best to think of vigorous exercise as being a *right or privilege* to which we are entitled for having 'paid our dues' (in terms of fitness); but it is not a necessity – and may actually be a hindrance – to becoming fit and healthy.

Here, bicycling, swimming – perhaps racquetball or soccer – would be the activities of choice . . . assuming they were pleasurable.

Keeping in mind that it is a privilege, not a requirement, of fitness to do strenuous exercise will help you also keep in mind the amount you are 'entitled' to (without injuring health). And if you have been over-indulgent in food or drink (for a short period of time – not chronically), a small (medicinal) amount of vigorous exercise can 'force' the liver – and subsequently the kidneys and other organs – to help the cleansing process move along quickly.

About fasting

Another technique which has many medicinal uses is *fasting*. A fast – which is a short-to-long avoidance of solid food – may be used for cleansing, temporary weight loss and/or spiritual discipline, depending on the length and type of fast undertaken.

A short fast – one which lasts approximately 24 hours – helps rid the body of excess moisture and is most useful in relieving *acute* disease (such as a cold, influenza, etc.). The body does not begin to lose 'stored' weight (in the form of fat) until about 48 hours after beginning a fast.

A 'deep cleansing fast' may last seven days or longer (possibly even a *month*, with careful supervision). This serves the purpose of ridding the body of accumulated 'toxins' (results of abusive practices). The cleansing fast is usually recommended – for at least a few days – before embarking on a 'mono-diet' (one that is used specifically for finding 'hidden' food allergies – see COOKING NATURALLY FOR PLEASURE AND HEALTH, or THE PULSE TEST, by Dr Arthur Coca, Arc Books, New York).

Fluids: vital when fasting

With the exception of the one day fast, it is vital to drink larger-than-normal quantities of fluids (preferably fresh water or freshly squeezed vegetable or fruit – but not citrus – juices). The reason that fluid intake must be carefully controlled is that the electrolytic balance of the body may be easily upset without sufficient liquids coming in.

The one exception to the 'no citrus' rule is *lemon juice.* Many natural health authorities recommend using lemon juice plus maple syrup (or as a less-preferable alternative, honey) and cayenne pepper (all diluted in a glass of water) for the *cleansing fast.* Here, the spicy lemonade is taken four or five times daily for up to several days in a row; the purpose is to stimulate the liver – a function which is normally accomplished by food – for blood purification.

Modified fasting for weight loss

A gentle way to fast for weight loss is the 'modified fast' – that is, to avoid a certain number of meals per week that you might ordinarily eat (e.g., skipping two lunches a week, but not 'making up for it' at dinner). This will promote a gradual weight loss and help the body to readjust to its lowering weight without undergoing the 'rubber ball' or *bounce-back* reaction that usually occurs following a 'crash diet'. It is quite possible to lose 30 or 40 pounds in a year – even more – by simply avoiding two or three meals a week.

But a fast – especially a long or deep-cleansing fast – should not be considered without your doctor's approval, especially if you've been suffering from serious health problems. This is of particular importance if you have been under – or are presently using – medication. A fast will help force residues from many chemical substances into the blood stream at a rapid rate, and if you are in poor or delicate health, you may create a 'healing crisis' of serious proportions. In any event, a doctor is always good to consult whenever you are considering *any* radical changes in your diet or healthstyle.

Review

Remember to do these practices each day:

* Stretching;
* Energy-balancing techniques;
* Deep breathing exercises – keep tongue tucked in the roof of the mouth;
* Rest frequently – take a siesta or mid-afternoon nap, if possible;
* Walk at least 300 or 400 steps daily (try to climb a flight or two of stairs in your walking), and do other gentle isotonic exercises;
* Meditative relaxation and visualization;
* Pleasure and play – enjoy yourself as much as possible;
* EAT RIGHT (eat *moderately*, regionally, seasonally – eat five or six *small* meals daily, with the largest consumed early in the day, and move toward a humane vegetarian diet, as quickly as

possible; *avoid abusive or allergenic foods and substances!*).

And do these techniques regularly – every day in the beginning of this program, then every several days, or so, as health and fitness are restored:

* The ten basic G-Jo isometric (no-movement or *static*) exercises;
* Moderate isotonic (movement) exercises, especially 'slow dance' and 'swinging arms', etc.;
* Self-massage (of the hands, feet, nose and scalp);
* G-Jo acupressure techniques, as needed;
* Acupressure eye exercises.

Finally, do the following *medicinally* or only occasionally:

* Vigorous exercising (enough to bring profuse perspiration);
* Fasting.

Follow this program faithfully and you will create for yourself a healthful and energy-filled life; the techniques are easy to both learn and remember . . . they require very little investment of time or energy . . . they're actually quite fun . . . and you'll feel wonderful after doing them. Best wishes for great health!

Section III:
Some Useful G-Jo Acupressure Point Illustrations

G-Jo Points which ease Aching Muscles

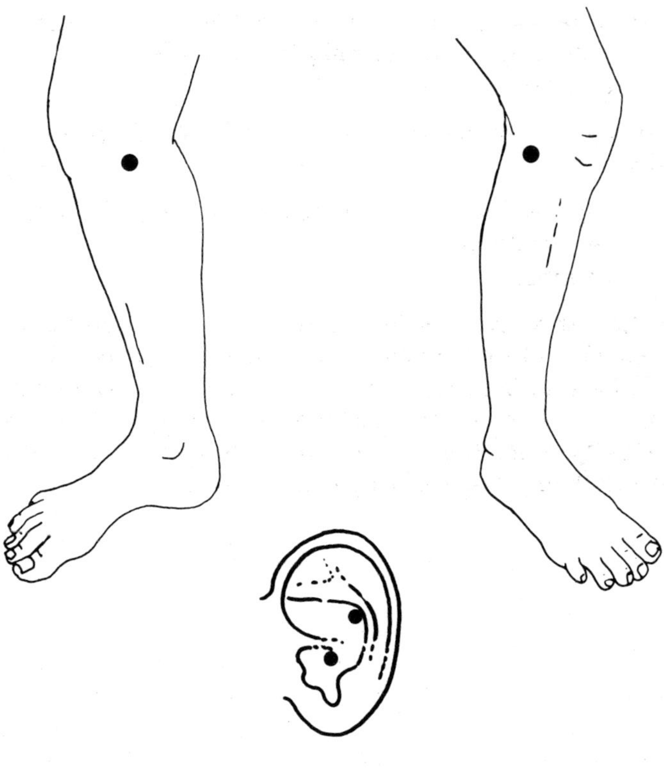

Muscle Relaxing Points

G-Jo Points which help Abdominal Development

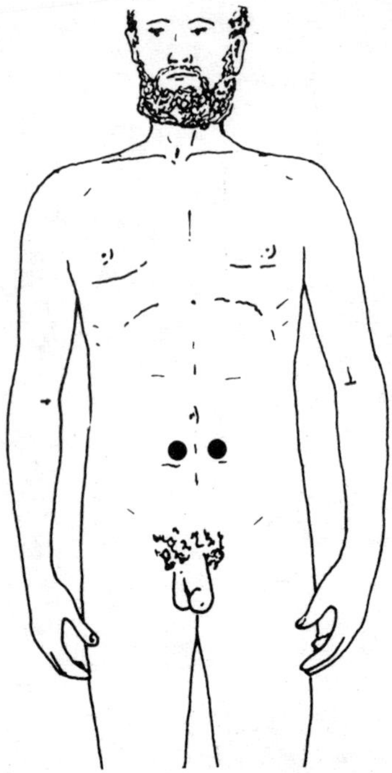

Abdominal Development Points

G-Jo Points which help relieve Stress and Tension and deepen Relaxation

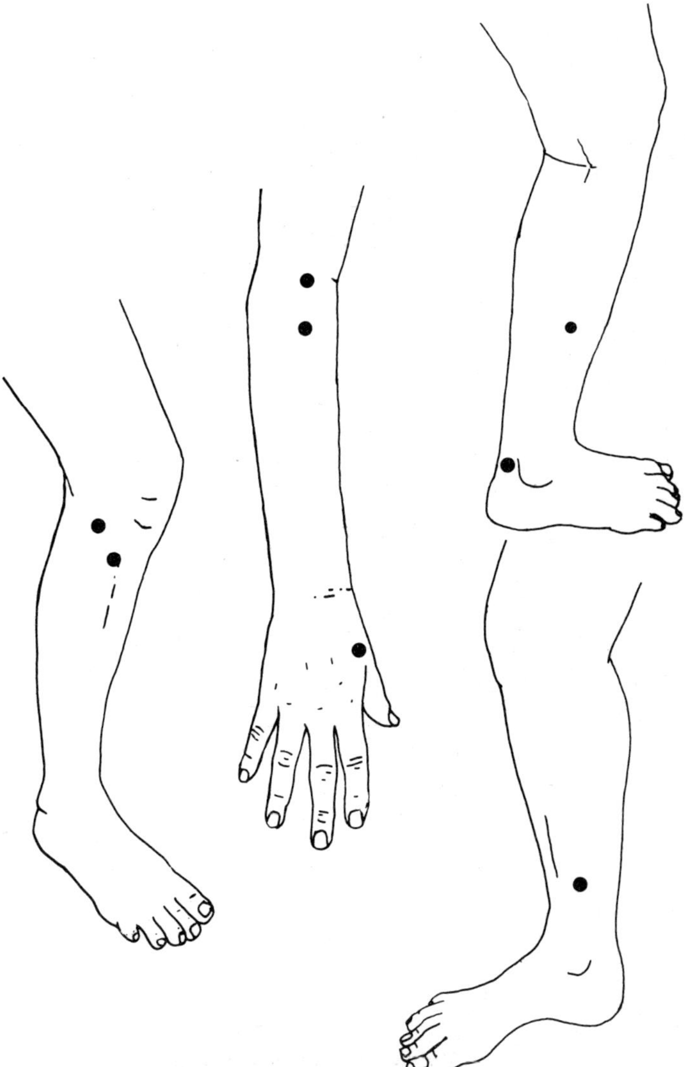

Some Useful G-Jo Acupressure Point Illustrations

Pain Relief Points

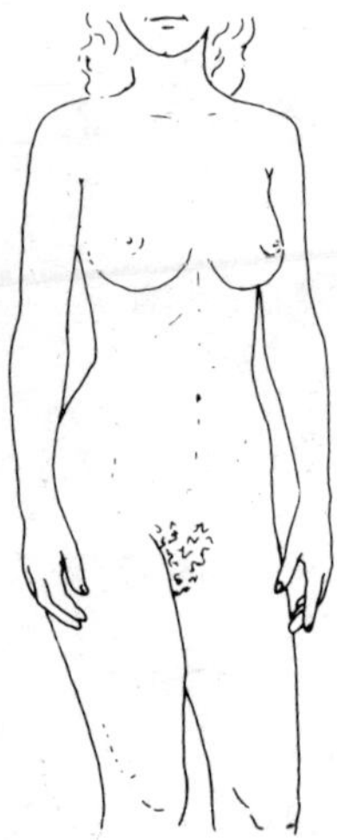

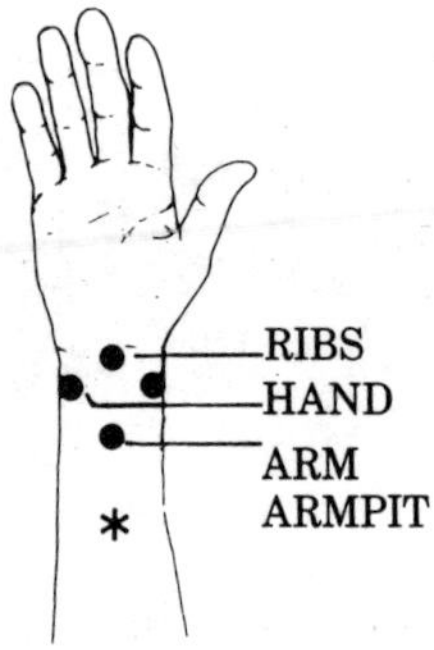

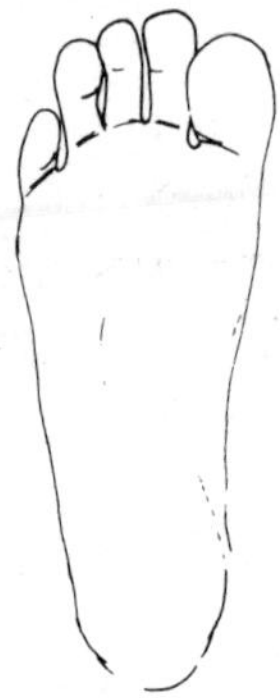

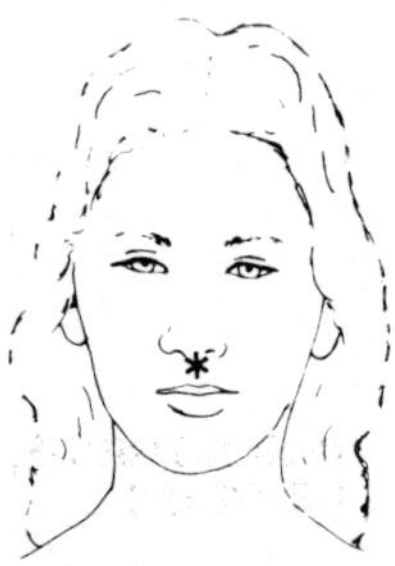

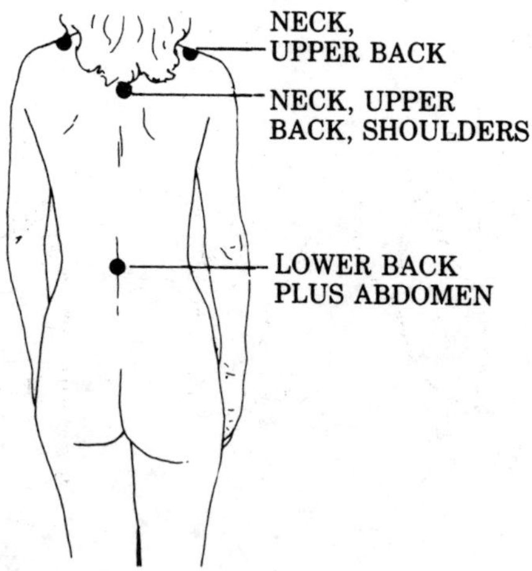

Pain Relief Points

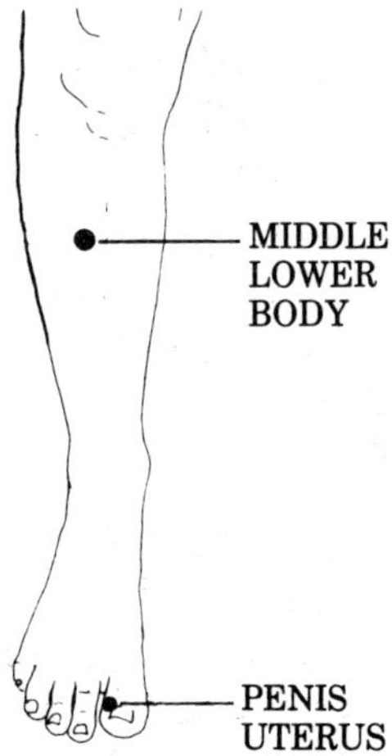

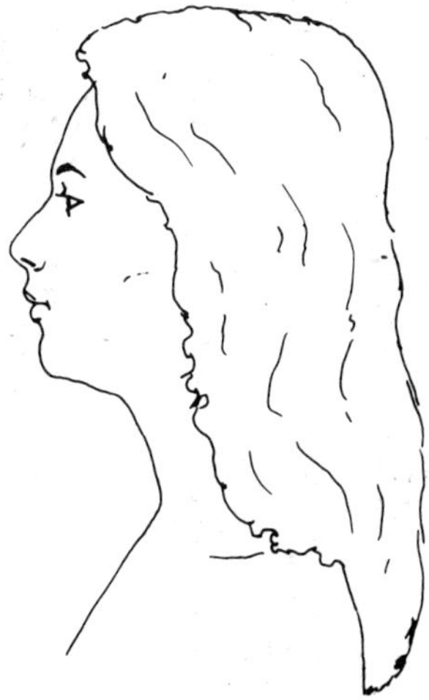

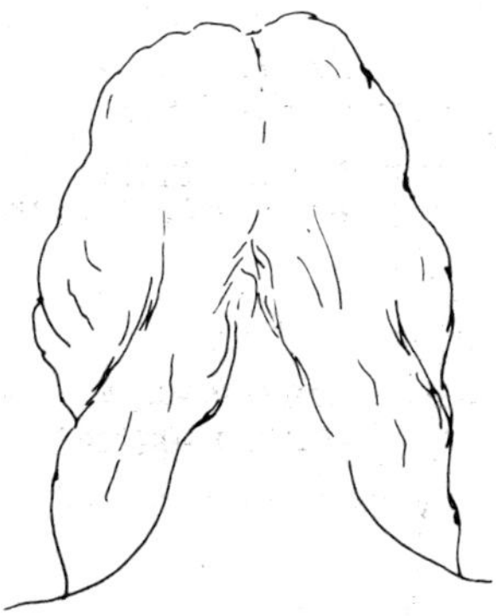

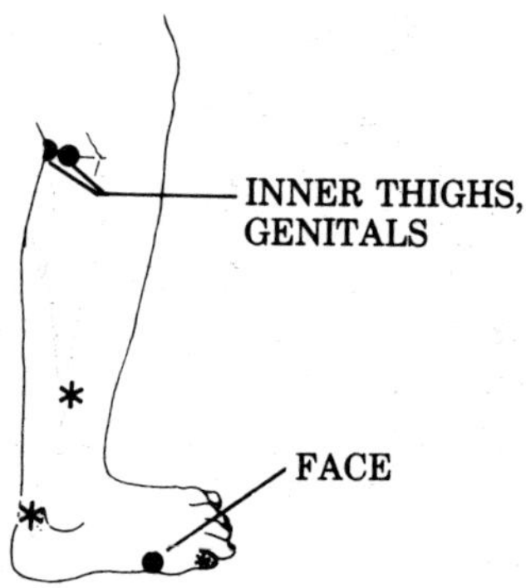

Some Useful G-Jo Acupressure Point Illustrations

Pain Relief Points

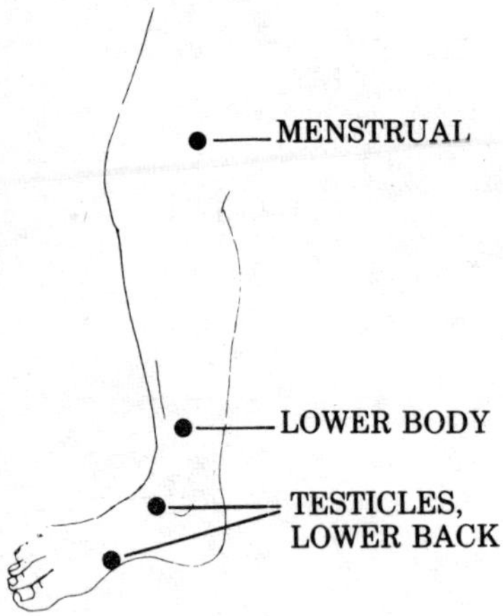

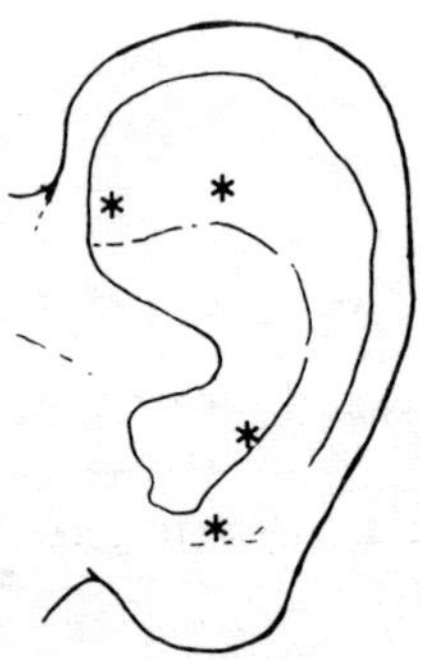

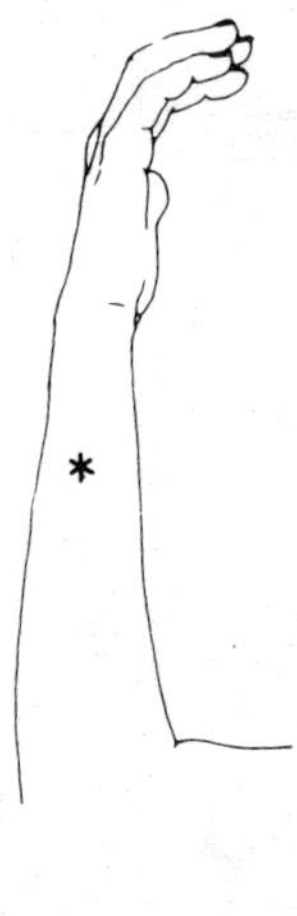

Pain Relief Points

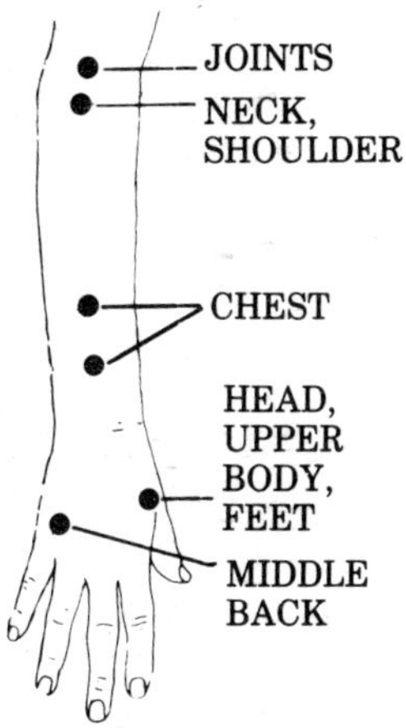

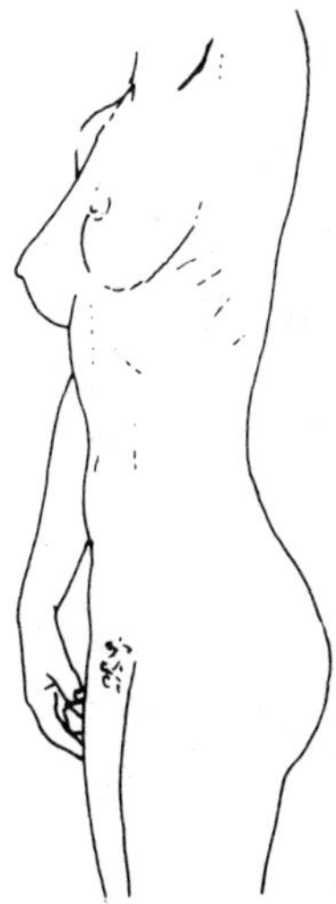

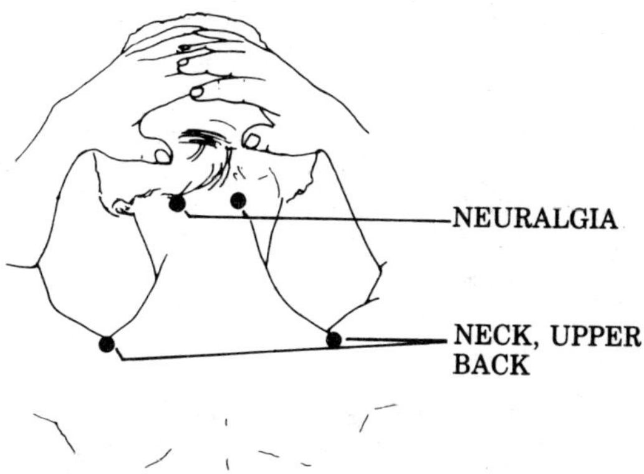

Some Useful G-Jo Acupressure Point Illustrations

The Chinese Acupressure Eye Exercises

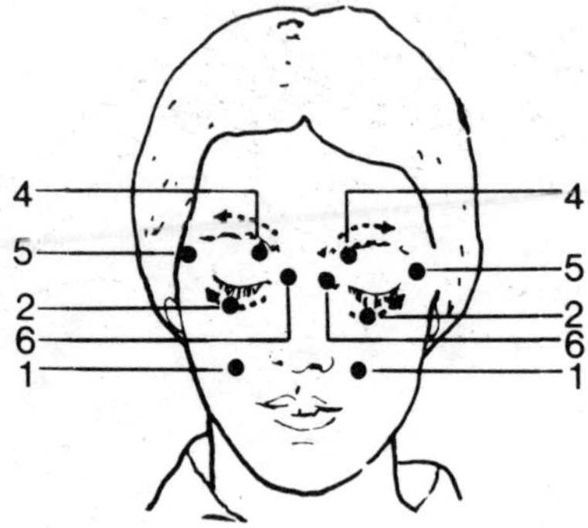

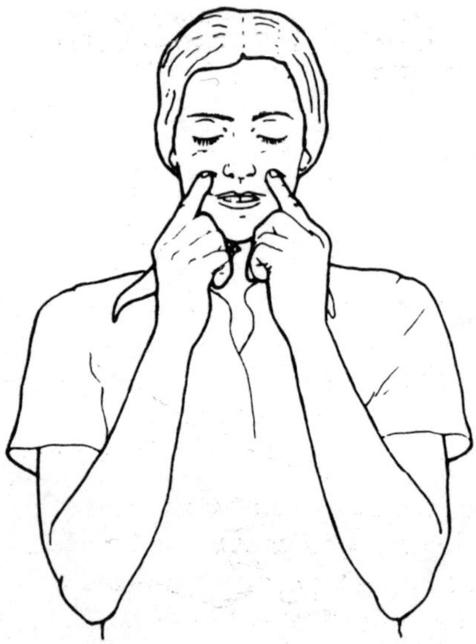

1. About the width of two fingers from the sides of the nostrils, in vertical line with the pupils.

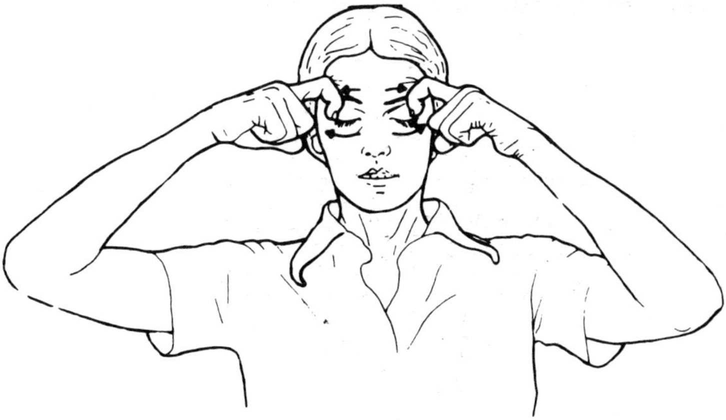

2. Along the inner edges of the eye sockets (top and bottom), drawn outwards, from the nose toward the temples.

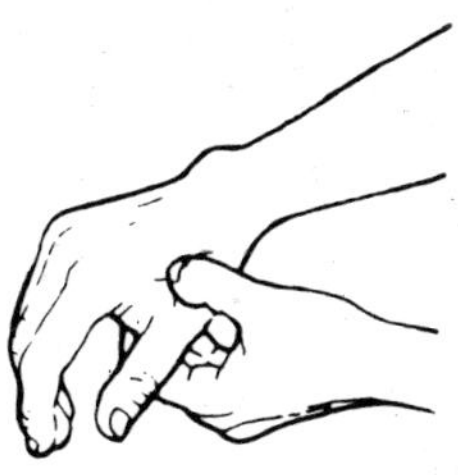

3. In the webbing, between the thumb and index finger on the back (top) of the hand.

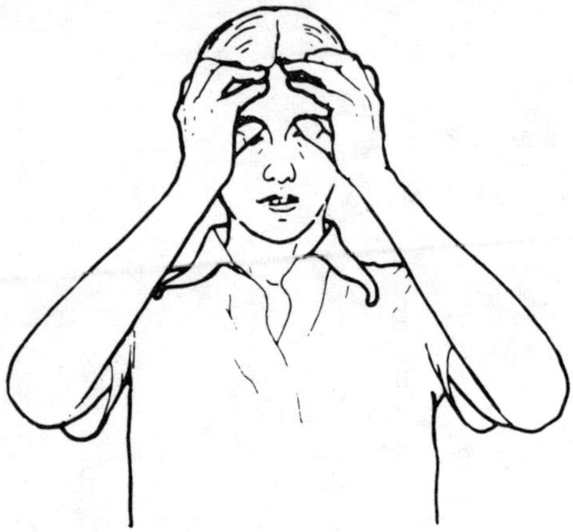

4. Under the inside corners of the eyebrows (best way to stimulate these is to put tips of fingers along hairline, tips of thumbs in the tender spots at inner corners of eye socket and massage like a 'spider doing pushups').

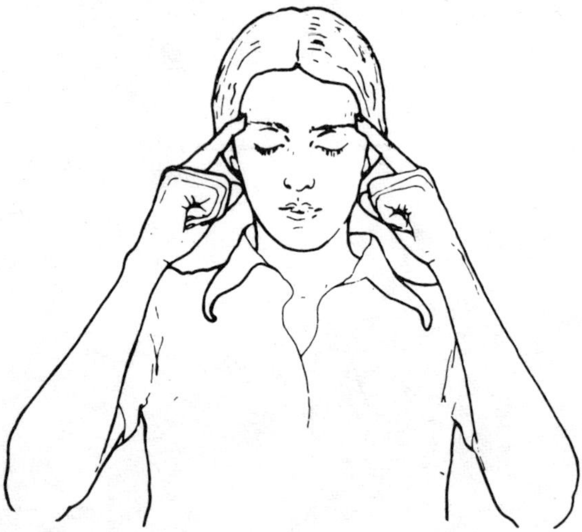

5. At the outer edges of the eyebrows, in the soft spots found there.

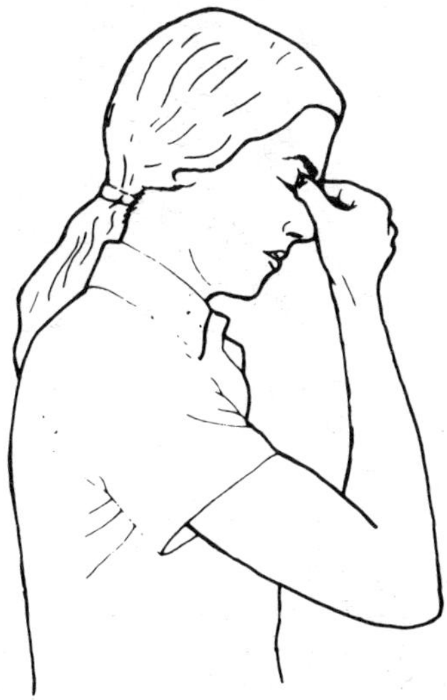

6. In the inner corners of the eye (cantharis).

Section IV:
Some Vegetarian Recipes For Fitness And Health

Following the delicious recipes and suggestions below, you will receive enough protein and other nutrients to maintain peak energy, while at the same time promoting gentle cleansing, weight loss (where necessary), and a humane, uplifted point of view. Many other delicious, healthful recipes will be found in COOKING NATURALLY FOR PLEASURE AND HEALTH: A WAY OF EATING.

Recipe Index

Fruits

Individual Fruits

Legumes

Nuts and seeds

Nuts

Seeds

Vegetables

Fruits

Individual Fruits

APPLE BAKE

4 baking apples
2 Tbsp. butter or soy margarine, melted
1 tsp. ground cinnamon
4 dried figs, chopped
8 dried apricots, chopped
½ cup raisins
¼ cup apple juice concentrate
¼ cup chopped walnuts

Wash and core the apples; leave ½ inch at the bottom. Combine the remaining ingredients and mix well. Spoon the stuffing into the cored apples and bake at 350°F. until tender, about 30 minutes. Serves 4.

(M)APPLE SYRUP

3 cups apple juice
1 cup maple syrup
½ cup apple juice concentrate
4 Tbsp. arrowroot
Pinch of sea salt
½ tsp. vanilla extract

Combine all the ingredients except the vanilla in a saucepan and bring to a boil. Reduce the heat and simmer until thickened, stirring continuously. Remove from the heat; stir in the vanilla and serve over waffles, pancakes or puddings. Makes 4½ cups.

APRICOT-NUT BREAD

½ cup apricot nectar or water

¼ cup maple syrup
½ cup chopped dried apricots
½ cup raisins
1½ cups whole wheat flour
2 tsp. low-sodium baking powder
½ tsp. baking soda
½ tsp. sea salt
2 eggs or equivalent egg replacer
¼ cup melted butter or soy margarine
1 Tbsp. cider or rice vinegar
1 tsp. vanilla extract
½ cup chopped walnuts

Preheat the oven to 350°F. In a medium saucepan, combine the apricot nectar, maple syrup, apricots and raisins. Bring to a boil; remove from the heat and cool. In a large mixing bowl, sift together the dry ingredients. Stir in the apricot mixture and the remaining ingredients and turn into an oiled 9-inch loaf pan. Bake for 40-45 minutes. Cool and serve. Makes 1 large loaf.

BANANA SHERBET

Peel overripe bananas (allow 1 banana per serving) and freeze overnight in a plastic bag. Chop into ½-inch pieces and blend in a food processor or blender until creamy. Add a little apple juice, if needed, to help blend. Serve in pretty parfait glass with a strawberry, sprig of mint or slice of orange and nuts as a garnish.

BLUEBERRY-OATMEAL WAFFLES

1 cup fresh or frozen blueberries
½-1 cup chopped pecans
4 cups oatmeal
¼ cup rice flour
1 tsp. *each* sea salt, ginger and cinnamon

4 cups milk, NUT MILK p. 124 or water
¼ cup cold-pressed oil *and* sweetener (maple or rice syrup, etc.)
1 Tbsp. lemon juice
2 tsp. vanilla extract

Set the blueberries and nuts aside. Mix the dry ingredients in a large bowl; stir in the milk. Combine the remaining ingredients and stir into the oatmeal mixture; refrigerate until thick, or prepare and refrigerate the night before. When ready to cook, fold in the blueberries and pecans; spoon the batter onto a preheated waffle iron and cook for 7-10 minutes. Serve with BLUEBERRY SAUCE (below). (M)APPLE SYRUP p. 76 or plain yogurt. Makes 8 waffles.

BLUEBERRY SAUCE

2 cups fresh or frozen unsweetened blueberries
½ cup apple juice
2 Tbsp. sweetener (maple or rice syrup, etc.)
2 Tbsp. arrowroot

Purée the blueberries in a food processor or blender. Pour into a saucepan with the remaining ingredients and bring to a boil. Reduce the heat and simmer, stirring continuously, until thickened. Serve on muffins, pancakes or waffles. Makes about 2 cups.

CHERRY BANANAS

1 Tbsp. butter or soy margarine
3 Tbsp. black cherry concentrate
4 medium bananas, cut diagonally into ½-inch chunks
1 cup pitted cherries
½ cup seltzer water
¼ cup black cherry concentrate
¼ tsp. ground cinnamon

1 Tbsp. arrowroot

Melt the butter in a saucepan; add the 3 Tbsp. black cherry concentrate, the bananas and the cherries and stir until well coated. Remove and set aside. Combine the remaining ingredients in the saucepan and bring to a boil; reduce the heat and simmer, stirring continuously until thickened. Pour over the bananas and cherries and serve warm or chilled. Serves 6.

CRANBERRY RELISH

1 cup cranberries, stemmed and finely chopped
1 apple, cored and finely chopped
$\frac{1}{4}$ cup water
$\frac{1}{4}$ cup frozen orange juice concentrate
$\frac{1}{4}$ cup frozen apple juice concentrate
1 Tbsp. agar-agar flakes

Combine all the ingredients in a small saucepan and boil gently for at least 5 minutes, stirring frequently. Set aside to cool. Refrigerate overnight to blend the flavors and serve cold on muffins, waffles, etc. or with nut or lentil loaves. Makes 2 cups.

DATE DIP OR STUFFING

8 oz. cream cheese or tofu
2 Tbsp. barley malt or maple syrup
$\frac{1}{8}$ tsp. ground cinnamon
$\frac{1}{8}$ tsp. ground cardamom
$\frac{1}{8}$ tsp. ground ginger
2 Tbsp. chopped raisins
2 Tbsp. chopped nuts
2 Tbsp. chopped dates

Mix all ingredients well. (If tofu is used, blend in a food processor or blender and add 2 additional Tbsp. syrup and a pinch of sea salt.) Use as a dip for sliced fruit and crackers or stuff into pitted dates. Makes about 1¼ cups.

GRAPE DELIGHT

1 lb. seedless green grapes
¼ cup maple or rice syrup
½ cup apple juice concentrate
A few drops rum extract
3 small cantaloupes, chilled
½ cup dairy sour cream or plain yogurt

Remove the stems from the grapes; combine with the syrup, apple juice concentrate and the rum extract. Chill for several hours, tossing occasionally. Cut the cantaloupes in half, scalloping the edges; scoop out the seeds. Toss the grapes with the yogurt or sour cream and spoon into the cantaloupes. Serves 6.

MELON PARFAIT

3 Tbsp. agar-agar flakes
½ cup pineapple juice
¼ cup *each* lime juice and orange juice concentrate
¼ cup rice syrup or maple syrup
½ cup seltzer water
2 cups *each* honeydew and cantaloupe balls
1 cup watermelon balls
1 cup strawberries, cut in half

In a small saucepan, dissolve the agar-agar flakes in the pineapple juice, lime juice, syrup and orange juice concentrate. Bring to a boil; reduce the heat and simmer for about 5 minutes, stirring continuously. Remove from the heat, add the seltzer water and chill until firm, about 2 hours. Meanwhile, prepare the melon balls and strawberries; cover and refrigerate for at least 1 hour. When ready to serve, beat the agar mixture with a fork.

Then spoon alternate layers of the agar mixture and fruit into parfait glasses. Top with a sprig of fresh mint. Serves 6.

ORANGE-TAPIOCA PUDDING

½ cup quick-cooking, granulated tapioca
¼ cup maple syrup
2 tsp. grated orange peel
½ tsp. *each* lemon extract and vanilla extract
Pinch of sea salt
2 cups NUT MILK p. 124
1 orange, peeled and cut into 8 slices

Combine all the ingredients except the orange slices in a small saucepan. Bring to a boil; reduce the heat and simmer for 10 minutes, stirring continuously. Cool slightly; pour into custard cups and top with an orange slice. Serve warm or chilled. Serves 8.

PEACH COBBLER

6 cups sliced fresh peaches *and* ½ cup peach nectar
1 cup oatmeal
⅓ cup ground pecans
¼ cup brown rice flour
1 tsp. ground cinnamon *and* a pinch of sea salt
¼ cup maple syrup
¼ cup raisins

Butter a pie plate; cover the bottom with the peaches and nectar. Combine the oatmeal, pecans, flour, cinnamon and syrup and mix well; sprinkle on the peaches, dot with butter, if desired, and bake until the peaches are soft. Top with ALMOND CREAM p. 120. Serves 8.

PEARS DELIGHT

3 large fresh pears, peeled
12 whole cloves
3 Tbsp. rice syrup or maple syrup
⅓ cup orange juice concentrate
1 Tbsp. lemon juice
1 stick cinnamon
1 apple, sliced
1 large orange, peeled and sliced thinly

Cut the pears in half lengthwise; press 2 cloves into the center of each half. Bring the syrup, orange concentrate, lemon juice and cinnamon stick to a boil in a large saucepan, stirring continuously; add the pears and apple slices to the syrup. Simmer uncovered, turning occasionally, until tender, for 10-15 minutes. Place the pears and apples in a serving dish; add the orange slices and top with the orange syrup. Serves 4.

PINEAPPLE-STRAWBERRY SHERBET

2 cups crushed pineapple, drained
6 oz. unsweetened pineapple juice concentrate
1 pint fresh strawberries, sliced
Fresh mint sprigs

Combine the pineapple and concentrate and blend until smooth; pour into a shallow container and freeze semi-hard. Whisk until smooth and slushy; fold in the sliced strawberries and freeze until firm. Garnish individual servings with fresh mint. Serves 4.

RAISIN-SPICE COOKIES

½ cup butter or soy margarine
¼ cup maple syrup
½ tsp. vanilla extract

1 egg or equivalent egg replacer
1¼ cups flour (rice, soy, unbleached, whole wheat)
1 cup oatmeal
¼ tsp. sea salt
½ tsp. low-sodium baking powder
½ tsp. *each* ground cinnamon, ginger and cardamom
½ cup *each* raisins and chopped nuts

Preheat oven to 350°F. Melt the butter; add the maple syrup, egg or egg replacer and vanilla and beat until creamy. Sift the flour, salt, baking powder and spices together and stir into the butter mixture. Then stir in the raisins and nuts and set aside for ½ hour. (If the batter is too dry, stir in just a little NUT MILK p. 124.) Drop by the teaspoonful onto an oiled cookie sheet, about 1 inch apart. Bake for about 15 minutes or until golden brown. Makes about 1½ dozen.

Fruit Combinations

CAROB-COATED FRESH FRUIT

Carob Coating:
¼ cup butter or soy margarine
¼ cup maple syrup
6 Tbsp. carob powder
¼ cup dairy, soy or NUT MILK p. 124
½ tsp. vanilla extract
Pinch of sea salt

Fruit:
4 ripe bananas, peeled and cut into 1-inch pieces
1 cup finely ground peanuts, optional
  or
2 pints fresh strawberries
  or
Other fresh fruit of choice

Melt the butter in a small saucepan. Add the maple syrup, carob powder, milk and salt; mix well and simmer for about 5 minutes, stirring continuously. Add the vanilla and stir well; set aside to cool. Dip each piece of fruit into the cooled carob mixture until well coated; roll the bananas in the ground peanuts. Place on wax paper or a buttered platter to set. If the kitchen is too warm for the carob to set properly, place in the refrigerator or freezer until ready to serve as a snack or dessert. Serves 8.

DRIED FRUIT COMPOTE

3 cups mixed dried fruit (figs, dates, raisins, etc.)
Cold water to cover fruit
2 Tbsp. agar-agar
Mace or cinnamon and fresh lemon juice to taste
¾ cup cooked BROWN RICE p. 92

Soak the dried fruit overnight in cold water. Then stew them in the same water with a touch of mace or cinnamon, until soft, about 20 minutes. Add the agar-agar and simmer 5 more minutes, stirring continuously. Mix in the rice and fresh lemon juice. Serve as a topping for pancakes or toast, or as a filling in pies or tarts. Makes about 4 cups.

DRIED FRUIT COOKIES

2 cups DRIED FRUIT COMPOTE (above)
½ cup butter or soy margarine, melted
¼ cup maple syrup
3 eggs or equivalent egg replacer
2 tsp. vanilla extract
2 cups cooked BROWN RICE p. 92
1½ cups brown rice flour
1 Tbsp. low-sodium baking powder

½ tsp. sea salt

Preheat the oven to 350°F. Blend the DRIED FRUIT COMPOTE in a blender or food processor and set aside. Combine the wet ingredients in a small bowl. In a large bowl, combine the dry ingredients; stir in the wet mixture. Drop by the heaped tablespoonful onto an oiled baking sheet; flatten to ½-inch thickness and spread the compote over the top. Bake for 20 minutes, until golden brown. Makes 1 dozen large cookies.

FRESH FRUIT PIE

Crust: BROWN RICE FLOUR PIE CRUST p. 92, baked

Filling:
½ cup frozen orange juice concentrate
2 cups pineapple juice
3 Tbsp. arrowroot or agar-agar flakes
Maple syrup or other sweetener to taste, optional (try a few dried figs or dates blended in the food processor with a little juice)
6 cups assorted fresh fruit, cut bite-sized — frozen, unsweetened fruit can also be used (raspberries, blueberries, strawberries, peaches, apples, pears, pineapple, etc.)
Shredded, unsweetened coconut and fresh mint

In a small saucepan, heat the orange and pineapple juices. Add the arrowroot or agar-agar and sweetener and boil gently for 5 minutes; remove from the heat and cool completely. Fold in the fresh fruit (drained) and turn into the baked crust. Garnish with coconut and fresh mint leaves. Serves 8.

FRESH FRUIT SMOOTHIES

In a blender or food processor, place the suggested fruit

combinations, or experiment with your own (note: peel overripe bananas before freezing in a plastic bag or freezer container). Add 1 Tbsp. unsweetened protein powder, if desired, and blend until smooth. Add crushed ice or seltzer water, and serve. Each combination makes about 1 cup.

1. ½ banana, frozen
   3 strawberries, frozen
   ½ cup apple juice

2. ½ cup skim milk or NUT MILK p. 124
   2 tsp. plain yogurt
   ½ tsp. vanilla
   ½ banana, papaya, peach or mango
   Cinnamon to taste

3. 1 cup unsweetened pineapple juice
   ½ banana, frozen

4. ½ cup orange juice
   ¼ cup grapefruit juice
   ½ cup fresh pineapple chunks
   A sprinkle of freshly grated coconut

5. ¼ cup apple juice concentrate
   ½ cup raspberries
   ¼ cup yogurt

6. ⅓ cup apple juice
   ⅓ cup apricot nectar
   4 fresh or presoaked, dried apricots
   ½ cored apple
   ½ tsp. vanilla

7. 1 cup orange juice
   1 Tbsp. cranberry concentrate
   1 tsp. lemon juice
   Pinch of cinnamon

8. 1 cup fresh pineapple chunks
   1 Tbsp. black cherry concentrate
   ¼ cup orange juice

9. 1 cup coconut milk
   1 medium peach
   2 Tbsp. plain yogurt
   ½ tsp. vanilla

Grains

General

ABOUT GRAINS

This section includes a few suggested dishes using whole or slightly processed grains. Because grains are the mainstay of a vegetarian diet, they are also suggested accompaniments to many non-grain recipes.

The less processing done to a grain, the greater its nutritional value. Therefore, whenever possible, use whole grains, and whenever practical, grind them to make your own cereals and flours. Combining whole grains and legumes (beans, peas, lentils) in a 2:1 ratio produces complete, balanced, usable proteins. In addition to providing extra nutritional value, flavor and texture to your meals, whole grains are relatively inexpensive and can be prepared in time- and energy-conserving ways. See the following cooking methods:

Presoaking: Presoaking the hard grains (whole wheat berries, hulled rye, oats, etc.) overnight or bringing to a boil, then soaking for 2 hours, will reduce the cooking time by about ⅓.

Regular Cooking: Wash the grains well in cold water. Place the water (refer to the GRAIN COOKING TIME CHART, p. 88 for the appropriate amount) in a heavy pot with tight-fitting lid; add salt, if desired, and bring to a boil. Stir in the grain and return to a boil. Cover, reduce the heat and simmer for the time suggested on the chart. (DO NOT stir again until ready to serve or the grains will become sticky). When the cooking time is up, turn off the heat and leave the pot on the cooking burner until ready to serve.

Pressure Cooking: Follow the same procedures as for

REGULAR COOKING up through the point of covering the pot. Then bring the pressure up 15lbs. and cook for the suggested time (see chart). When the cooking time is up, cool immediately under water to release the pressure; cover again and set aside, away from the heat, until ready to serve.

Or: Place 1 or 2 inches of water in the bottom of a pressure cooker. Place the measured grain in a stainless steel bowl inside the cooker and add water to fill the bowl about $\frac{3}{4}$ to 1 inch above the grain. Cover, then continue the pressure-cooking process. (This is a good way to cook beans and grains at the same time — beans on the bottom, grains in the bowl, on top.)

Thermos Cooking: *For rolled or cracked grains* — preheat a wide-mouth thermos bottle (fill it with hot water and empty just before using). Fill the preheated thermos $\frac{1}{4}$ full with any rolled or cracked grain. Then pour in boiling water $\frac{3}{4}$ full; close tightly and lay the thermos on its side for 8-10 hours. Open when ready to serve.

GRAIN COOKING TIME CHART

One cup of grain (unsoaked)	**Amount of water**	**Regular cooking time**	**Pressure cooker time**
Rolled, flaked or cracked grain (oatmeal, cracked wheat, rye, etc.)	2 cups	5–10 min.	—
Parboiled or soft grains (bulgur, buckwheat, kasha, millet)	$2\frac{1}{2}$ cups	20 min.	10 min.
Medium whole grains (hulled barley, brown rice)	2 cups	40–55 min.	30 min.
Hard whole grains (oats, rye, triticale, wheat berries)	$2\frac{1}{2}$ cups	1–$1\frac{1}{2}$ hrs.	45 min.

NOTES TO GRAIN COOKING TIME CHART

1. Rolled flakes or cracked grains are *not recommended for pressure cooking* because of their tendency to clog the steam vent.
2. The amount of water and length of cooking time will vary, depending on the source of heat and type of cooking pot used; adjust accordingly.
3. For pressure cooking: the amount of water used may be reduced slightly when cooking more than one cup of a grain — but there is no specific ratio. Experiment with the different grains in your specific situation.

BASIC GRANOLA

Basic Recipe:
¼ cup cold-pressed oil
¼ cup maple syrup
½ tsp. vanilla extract
3 cups oatmeal
¼ tsp. sea salt
½ cup chopped nuts
½ cup raisins or chopped fruit

Dry Ingredients:
Flaked oats, wheat, rye, soy, corn, etc.; seeds; wheat germ and other brans; powdered milk; salt, cinnamon, ginger, lemon peel and other spices; chopped almonds, cashews, pecans, walnuts or other nuts.

Wet Ingredients:
Cold-pressed oil; melted butter or soy margarine; maple syrup; fruit juice concentrates; molasses; rice syrup; barley malt; vanilla extract.

Fruit:
Shredded coconut; raisins; chopped dried dates, apples, figs, apricots, pineapple, prunes, etc.

Use the BASIC RECIPE and add any of the alternative dry and wet ingredients, keeping a ratio of 6 cups dry ingredients to 1 cup wet ingredients and 1 cup fruit. Combine the wet ingredients in one bowl and the dry in another; mix each well. Then combine, mix and roast in a shallow pan at 250°F. for 30 minutes. After roasting, add the dried fruit. The basic recipe makes 4 cups.

Note: For a pie crust, press granola into a pie plate. If too dry, add a little fruit juice or melted butter; then fill and bake.

BREAD PUDDING

4 cups whole grain bread, cubed small
1 cup grated apples
½ cup golden raisins
3 cups NUT MILK p. 124
¼ tsp. ground cinnamon
⅛ tsp. *each* ground mace and nutmeg
1 Tbsp. *each* grated orange peel and molasses
2 Tbsp. melted butter
¼ cup maple or rice syrup or more to taste
2 eggs or equivalent egg replacer
1 tsp. vanilla extract

Place the bread cubes, grated apple and raisins in an oiled baking dish. Combine the remaining ingredients and whisk together well; stir into the bread mixture. Bake at 350°F. for 1 hour until set. Serves 8.

HARDY GRAIN PANCAKES

2 cups oatmeal, cooked
3 cups BROWN RICE p. 92, cooked

To Cook the Oatmeal:
Place 1¼ cups uncooked oatmeal in a wide-mouth, 1-quart thermos bottle. Pour in enough boiling water to fill and stir. Close the thermos and lay it on its side. In the morning the oatmeal will be thick and sticky and ready to use for pancakes.

To Make the Pancakes:
Mix the oatmeal and rice together well, forming a sticky ball; divide into 4 parts. Press each part into the bottom of a non-stick skillet to form a large, ½-inch thick pancake. Cook on medium-high heat, until both sides are crisp (about 30 minutes); flip often to keep from

burning. Serve with butter and (M)APPLE SYRUP p. 76. Makes 4 large pancakes.

Individual Grains

BARLEY-MUSHROOM SOUP

2-3 stalks celery, cut into 1-inch pieces
3 carrots, cut into 1-inch pieces
1 lb. mushrooms, sliced
1 cup barley, uncooked
2½ quarts vegetable stock or water
Sea salt or tamari and freshly ground pepper to taste

In a covered pot, steam the celery, carrots and ⅓ of the mushrooms until tender; then purée in a food processor, adding vegetable stock as needed. Sauté the rest of the mushrooms until tender in a large pot. Add the vegetable purée, the rest of the stock and the barley; season to taste. Cook on low heat about 1½ hours. Garnish with chopped parsley and serve. Serves 8.

BARLEY-VEGETABLE BURGERS

2 cups *each* cooked barley and millet
½ cup brown rice flour
¼ cup chopped onion, optional
½ cup *each* chopped celery, cooked green peas
½ cup grated carrots
¼ cup NUT BUTTER p. 123 (peanut, cashew, tahini)
2 Tbsp. tamari *and* ¼ tsp. dried basil
Sea salt and freshly ground pepper to taste

Combine all the ingredients in a large bowl and knead well; form into patties and bake at 350°F. for 20 minutes. Serve with MISO GRAVY p. 112. Makes 8-10 burgers.

Note: for 2 cups cooked grains, cook ¾ cup raw barley to 3½ cups water for 35-40 minutes and ¾ cup raw millet to 2 cups water for 20 minutes.

BROWN RICE

2 cups brown rice
4 cups water

Rinse the brown rice well; drain and set aside. Bring the water to a boil in a large saucepan. Add the rice, stir once (do not stir again or it will become sticky). Cover, reduce the heat and simmer for 55 minutes (until the water is absorbed). Turn off the heat and let the cooked rice sit on the warm burner until ready to serve. (For variety, substitute tomato juice, fruit juice or vegetable bouillon for the water.) Makes about 5 cups.

BROWN RICE CREAM CEREAL

¼ cup homemade cream of rice (instructions below)
1½ cups water (and pinch of salt, optional)
2 Tbsp. currants
⅓ cup cooked BROWN RICE (above)

To Prepare the Cream of Rice:
Place 2 cups of uncooked brown rice in a heavy skillet. Toast on medium-high heat until lightly browned, stirring constantly. Cool and grind in a Vita-Mix® or grain grinder to a fine powder. Store in a covered jar to use as a cereal or to thicken soups and sauces.

To Cook the Cereal:
Bring the water and salt to a boil; slowly stir in 3 Tbsp. of the cream of rice. Lower the heat and simmer for about 15 minutes, stirring frequently. Add the currants and brown rice. (A sweetener and/or NUT MILK p. 124 can be added, if desired.) Serves 1.

BROWN RICE FLOUR PIE CRUST

3 cups brown rice flour (or half rice and half wheat flour)
½ tsp. ground cinnamon
½ cup butter or soy margarine, melted
1 tsp. vanilla extract
½ cup finely ground almonds

1 Tbsp. maple syrup
1 cup ice cold water

Preheat the oven to 400°F. Sift the flour and cinnamon together in a large bowl. Add the almonds and cut in the butter until crumbly. Add the vanilla, maple syrup and a little water; knead with your fingers. Add the remaining water until a ball is formed. Knead 1 minute more. Sprinkle a pastry sheet or waxed paper with a little flour. Roll out half the dough into a circle about ⅛-inch thick and turn over into a buttered pie plate. (Rice flour dough will be dry and crumbly compared to wheat.) If the dough breaks when turning into the pan, just pat it together with your fingers and proceed. Crimp the edges and puncture the sides and center with a fork. Bake for 15 minutes or until the crust is golden brown. Freeze the other half of the dough or make 2 pies. Makes 2 crusts.

BROWN RICE-MUSHROOM RING

½ lb. mushrooms, sliced
½ cup chopped onions
2 Tbsp. butter or soy margarine
2 cups cooked BROWN RICE p. 92
½ cup slivered, blanched almonds, roasted
Sea salt, pepper and lemon juice to taste

Sauté the mushrooms and onions in the butter; add the remaining ingredients, adjust the seasoning and heat thoroughly. Press the mixture firmly into a buttered ring mold and let stand for about 5 minutes. Invert the rice mold on a platter and fill the center with buttered, steamed vegetables. Serves 4.

BROWN RICE PUDDING

3 cups cooked BROWN RICE p. 92
½ cup seedless raisins
½ cup apple juice
2 cups NUT MILK p. 124

¼ cup NUT BUTTER p. 123
Finely grated rind of 1 lemon
½ tsp. ground nutmeg
2-3 Tbsp. sweetener (rice, barley or maple syrup)
1 tsp. molasses
2 eggs or equivalent egg replacer
½ tsp. vanilla extract
⅛ tsp. sea salt

Place the rice and raisins in a mixing bowl and set aside. Combine the remaining ingredients in a blender or food processor and blend well. Stir into the rice mixture and pour into an oiled baking dish. Bake at 325°F. for 1 hour or until lightly browned. Serve with (M)APPLE SYRUP p. 76. Serves 8.

BROWN RICE-STUFFED CABBAGE

Cabbage Leaves:
Core a head of cabbage so that the outer leaves separate easily; steam for about 10-15 minutes until tender. Carefully peel off the leaves and blanch in boiling water for 5 minutes; drain. Plunge into cold water and fill with stuffing.

Stuffing:
1 cup textured vegetable protein (soy granules)
1 tsp. powdered vegetable broth
1 cup vegetable stock or water
1 small onion, chopped
¼ cup cold-pressed oil
1½-2 cups cooked BROWN RICE p. 92
2 Tbsp. chopped fresh parsley
1 tsp. paprika
⅛ tsp. garlic powder
⅛ tsp. dried basil or thyme
⅛ tsp. cayenne pepper
Sea salt to taste
1 cup chopped walnuts

Soak the textured vegetable protein in the powdered broth and stock or water and set aside. Sauté the onion; add the textured vegetable protein and the remaining ingredients. Mix well and adjust the seasoning to taste. Spoon the stuffing onto each cabbage leaf at the stem end and fold into a closed packet; place close together, seam down, in an oiled baking dish and dot with butter.

Sauce:
2 cups or more stewed tomatoes
½ cup chopped onion
2 Tbsp. butter or soy margarine
½ tsp. *each* dried basil and paprika
⅛ tsp. garlic powder
⅛ tsp. cayenne pepper
Squeeze of fresh lemon
½ cup or more sour cream or yogurt
Tamari or sea salt to taste

Combine all the sauce ingredients in a food processor and purée. Pour the sauce over the cabbage rolls and bake at 350°F. until the leaves are tender and sauce is bubbly (about 45 minutes). Serves 6-8.

BROWN RICE WAFFLES

2 cups cooked BROWN RICE p. 92
1½ cups brown rice flour
½ cup unbleached or whole wheat flour
½ tsp. *each* ground cinnamon, ginger and sea salt
½-1 cup chopped pecans
3 cups buttermilk
½ cup cold-pressed oil
¼ cup maple syrup
2 ripe bananas, mashed
1 tsp. vanilla extract

Combine all the dry ingredients in a large mixing bowl and set aside. In another bowl, combine the wet ingredients (including the bananas) and beat with a whisk until well blended; stir into the dry mixture to form a thick batter. Spoon onto the waffle iron and bake for about 8 minutes each. Makes 8 waffles.

BULGUR CASSEROLE

2 Tbsp. cold-pressed oil
½ cup chopped green onions
2 cups cooked corn kernels
2 cups cooked carrots, cut julienne-style
½ tsp. dried marjoram
3 Tbsp. chopped fresh parsley
1 Tbsp. powdered vegetable broth
4 cups vegetable stock or water
1½ cups bulgur
Sea salt and pepper to taste

In a large skillet, sauté the onions in the oil until tender. Stir in the corn, carrots and herbs; simmer for 5 minutes. In a large casserole dish, dissolve the powdered broth in the water and add the bulgur. Stir in the sautéed vegetables and adjust the seasoning. Cover and bake for 20 minutes at 350°F. Serves 8.

BULGUR PILAF

⅓ cup butter or soy margarine
⅔ cup vermicelli
4 cups water
Sea salt
2 cups coarse bulgur
Freshly ground pepper

In a saucepan melt the butter; add the vermicelli and sauté until lightly browned. Add the water and salt and bring to a boil. Stir in the bulgur; reduce the heat and simmer until water is absorbed. Toss with steamed or sautéed, chopped vegetables of choice; sprinkle with pepper and serve. Serves 6-8.

CORN MUFFINS

3 cups corn meal
1 Tbsp. low-sodium baking powder
1 tsp. baking soda
¼ tsp. sea salt
¼ cup melted butter or soy margarine
1 cup *each* buttermilk and hot water
3 Tbsp. apple juice concentrate

Preheat the oven to 400°F. Combine the dry ingredients and mix well; cut in the butter. Stir in the buttermilk and apple juice concentrate; add the hot water to make a soupy batter. Pour into oiled tins (¾ full) and bake for 15-20 minutes. Makes 1½ dozen.

CORN SALAD

4 cups cooked kernels
1 cup chopped celery
1 cup cooked green peas
½ cup chopped sweet red pepper
¼ cup chopped green onions, optional
¼ cup lemon juice
1 Tbsp. rice vinegar
⅓ cup olive oil
1 Tbsp. minced parsley
½ tsp. *each* dried basil and powdered vegetable broth
Sea salt and freshly ground pepper to taste

Combine all the vegetables in a large mixing bowl and toss. Place the remaining dressing ingredients in a screw-top jar and shake well. Pour over the vegetables and toss again. Chill well before serving on a bed of lettuce. Serves 6.

KASHA HOMESTYLE

2½ cups salted water
1½ cups diced potatoes
1 cup whole groats or coarse kasha (roasted buckwheat)
¼ cup butter or soy margarine
¼ cup green peas
¼ cup chopped sweet red pepper
2 green onions, sliced
¼ cup liquid soy protein
1 tsp. dried summer savory
Paprika
Yogurt, optional

Bring the water and potatoes to a boil in a saucepan and cook for 5 minutes. Add the kasha; reduce the heat and simmer for 10-15 minutes until the water is absorbed. In a large skillet, sauté the peas, pepper and green onions in the butter until tender. Stir in the liquid soy protein, savory and kasha mixture; fry like hash browns for 20 minutes. Sprinkle with paprika and serve with yogurt, if desired. Serves 4-6.

KASHA-RICE CEREAL

1½ cups water
¼ cup whole or coarse kasha (roasted buckwheat)
½ cup uncooked brown rice
⅛ tsp. sea salt, optional
¼ cup *each* raisins and chopped dates
NUT MILK p. 124 to taste

Bring the water to a boil. Add the kasha, brown rice, and salt; cover and simmer for 1 hour, until the water is absorbed. Mix in the raisins, dates and NUT MILK and serve. Serves 2.

MILLET-FRUIT PUDDING

1 quart NUT MILK p. 124
¼ cup sweetener (rice or maple syrup, barley malt)
¼ tsp. sea salt or to taste
1 tsp. *each* vanilla extract and fresh lemon juice
½ tsp. grated lemon or orange peel
1 cup raw millet
½ cup mixed dried fruit, chopped
¼ cup *each* raisins and grated unsweetened coconut
Dash of ground cinnamon

In a food processor or blender, process the NUT MILK, sweetener, salt, vanilla, lemon juice and peel; place in a saucepan with the millet and bring to a boil. Reduce heat; simmer for 15 minutes. Stir in the remaining ingredients and pour into a baking dish. Cover and bake for 1 hour at 350°F.; serve with (M)APPLE SYRUP p. 76. Serves 6-8.

MILLET MUFFINS

2 cups millet flour (ground raw millet)
1½ cups brown rice flour
1 Tbsp. low-sodium baking powder
½ tsp. baking soda
¼-½ tsp. sea salt, optional
2 Tbsp. melted butter or soy margarine
1 cup *each* buttermilk and hot water
2 Tbsp. sweetener (maple or rice syrup)

Preheat the oven to 400°F. Sift together the dry ingredients; cut in the butter. Combine the buttermilk and sweetener and stir into the dry mixture. Slowly add the hot water until the mixture is fluffy but a little soupy. Pour into oiled muffin tins (¾ full) and bake for 15 minutes. Makes 1½ dozen.

OATMEAL-FRUIT BARS

1 cup apple juice
½ cup butter or soy margarine, melted
¼ cup maple syrup
¼ cup apple juice concentrate
3 eggs or equivalent egg replacer
2 tsp. vanilla extract
2½ cups oatmeal
1 cup flour (unbleached, whole wheat, soy, rice, etc.)
3 tsp. low-sodium baking powder
½ tsp. sea salt
½ cup chopped nuts
½ cup raisins
1 cup combined dried dates, apricots, and apples, chopped

Preheat the oven to 325°F. Combine the wet ingredients in a small bowl and set aside. In a large mixing bowl, combine the remaining ingredients; add the wet mixture and stir well. Spread in a rectangular baking pan and bake for 30-35 minutes. Cool before cutting into squares. Makes 3 dozen squares.

OATMEAL WITH CINNAMON AND BANANAS

Prepare the oatmeal as directed for the quantity desired. (Or make in a thermos bottle: see HARDY GRAIN PANCAKES p. 90.) When the oatmeal is cooked, stir in ⅛ tsp. cinnamon per serving and top with sliced bananas and 1 tsp. chopped nuts. Add a little fruit juice concentrate or maple syrup for sweetener and NUT MILK p. 124, if desired.

WHEATBERRY CEREAL

1 cup wheatberries
2 cups water
¼ cup raisins

Sweetener to taste (rice or maple syrup, barley malt, molasses, fruit juice concentrate)
1 Tbsp. chopped walnuts
1 tsp. sunflower seeds
Sliced fruit, berries or chopped dried fruit

Place the wheatberries, water and raisins in a crock pot and cook overnight on low heat or cook in a pressure cooker for 40 minutes. When the berries are tender, drain the liquid, stir in the remaining ingredients and serve with NUT MILK p. 124, if desired. Serves 2.

WHOLE WHEAT DOUGHNUTS

1⅓ cups warm water
1 Tbsp. yeast
4 cups flour (½ whole wheat and ½ unbleached)
1 tsp. sea salt
2 Tbsp. sweetener (maple syrup, apple juice concentrate, molasses, barley malt, rice syrup)
¼ cup cold-pressed oil

Combine all the ingredients and mix just enough to moisten. Place the dough on an oiled surface and roll out to ½-inch thickness. Cut with a doughnut cutter and place on an oiled cookie sheet. Allow to rise and bake at 375°F. for 15-20 minutes. Serve with a sweet dipping sauce. Makes 2½ dozen.

Legumes

General

DRIED LEGUMES

When cooking dried beans, a pressure cooker conserves much time and energy. If you don't own a pressure cooker, follow the cooking instructions on the package.

To pressure-cook dried beans, the following general rules are important to keep in mind:

1. Allow 6 cups water to 2 cups dried beans and 2 Tbsp. cold-pressed oil (the oil coats the surface, preventing loose bean skins from clogging the steam vent).
2. If the steam vent clogs, remove the cooker from the heat and release the pressure; open and clean out the vent pipe. Then resume cooking.
3. Never fill the pressure cooker over ½ full.
4. DO NOT pressure-cook split peas, as they produce a foam which clogs up the steam vent.
5. Always follow the instructions in your pressure cooker manual.

Presoaking overnight and rinsing well before cooking substantially cuts down on the cooking time and aids the digestibility of the beans. If presoaking in a warm kitchen, refrigerate so that the beans will not sour or ferment. Skim off the floating skins prior to cooking. To make a bean gravy or soup, add more water, if necessary, to cover the beans and continue cooking for 15-30 minutes longer without the lid. Season to taste and add vegetables or use in other recipes.

Pressure cooking times for commonly used beans are listed in the following table:

LEGUME COOKING TIMES

Name of dried bean	**Pressure cooking times**	
	soaked	**unsoaked**
Black beans	35 min.	45–50 min.
Black-eyed peas	20 min.	30 min.

Garbanzo beans (chickpeas)	30 min.	1 hr.–1 hr., 15 min.
Great Northern beans	10-12 min.	30 min.
Kidney beans	25-30 min.	1 hr.–1 hr., 15 min.
Lentils	20 min.	30 min.
Lima beans	25 min.	1 hr.–1 hr., 15 min.
Navy beans	10-12 min.	25 min.
Pink beans	30 min.	1 hr.–1 hr., 15 min.
Pinto beans	25-30 min.	1 hr.–1 hr., 15 min.
Soybeans	30-40 min.	45 min.–1 hr.

Beans

EASY BEAN SALAD

2 cups fresh green beans, cooked tender-crisp
2 cups kidney beans, cooked
2 cups fresh wax beans, cooked tender-crisp
1 Tbsp. minced fresh parsley or 2 tsp. dried parsley
1 tsp. minced fresh basil or ½ tsp. dried basil
1 tsp. minced fresh oregano or ½ tsp. dried oregano
1 tsp. dried mustard
3 Tbsp. apple juice concentrate
1 Tbsp. rice vinegar
¼ cup lemon juice
⅓ cup olive oil
Sea salt and freshly ground pepper to taste

Place all the beans in a large mixing bowl. Combine the remaining ingredients in a screw-top jar and shake well; pour over the beans and toss. Chill well before serving in a bed of lettuce. Serves 4-6.

GARBANZO SALAD

2 Tbsp. olive oil
3 Tbsp. rice vinegar
Pinch of sea salt
3 cups cooked garbanzo beans (chickpeas)
6 red radishes
1 small cucumber
2 stalks celery
½ cup watercress
1 Tbsp. fresh parsley, finely chopped
2 tsp. fresh mint, chopped or 1 tsp. dried mint
1 pint alfalfa sprouts or lettuce
8 black olives
Watercress

Combine the oil, vinegar and salt; toss into the chickpeas and marinate overnight. About an hour before serving, slice and dice the vegetables to the size of the chickpeas. Stir into the chickpeas along with the parsley and mint. Place the salad on a bed of sprouts or lettuce and garnish with olives and whole watercress. Serve with pita bread.

ITALIAN BEAN STEW

4 cups macaroni
4 cups cooked navy or Great Northern beans
1 *each* carrot, celery stalk and potato, diced
½ cup chopped onion, optional
1 cup green beans, cut into ½-inch pieces
1 zucchini or yellow squash, chopped
1 Tbsp. chopped fresh parsley

2 tsp. mixed Italian herbs
2 cups *each* tomato sauce and vegetable stock
1 tsp. powdered vegetable broth
Tamari or sea salt and freshly ground pepper to taste
Grated Parmesan cheese, optional

Combine all the ingredients, except the macaroni, in a large soup pot and bring to a boil; simmer gently for 30 minutes, stirring occasionally, until the vegetables are tender. Add the macaroni and simmer 15 more minutes. Serve with Parmesan cheese. Serves 6-8.

LIMA BEANS AND KALE

2 lb. fresh kale, chopped (or 2 10-oz. pkg. frozen)
3 cups fresh or frozen or 2 cups dried lima beans
1 Tbsp. powdered vegetable broth
2-3 Tbsp. butter or soy margarine, optional
Herb seasoning salt and freshly ground pepper to taste

Cook the beans as directed until soft. Steam the kale until tender. (Reserve the liquid from both to use as vegetable stock.) Dissolve the powdered broth and butter in 1 cup of the reserved stock. Combine the cooked beans, kale and seasoned water and mix well; season to taste and serve with rice. Serves 4-6.

MIXED BEAN SOUP

½ cup *each* of six different dried beans (pinto, kidney, navy, lima, garbanzo, Great Northern, adzuki or black beans)
1½ quarts water for soaking
5 cups vegetable stock or water for cooking
½ cup chopped sweet red peppers
½ cup sliced celery
½ cup sliced carrots
1 clove garlic, minced, optional

1 bay leaf
1 tsp. dried basil
½ tsp. dried summer savory
¼ tsp. chili powder
2 Tbsp. tamari or ¼ cup liquid soy protein
¼ white wine, optional
1 Tbsp. powdered vegetable broth
½ cup barley
1 cup chopped tomatoes
½ tsp. sea salt, optional
2-3 Tbsp. butter or soy margarine

Rinse the beans well and soak overnight in 1½ quarts of water. When ready to cook, rinse again and drain; cook until tender (see DRIED LEGUMES p. 101). Add the remaining ingredients and pressure-cook or simmer until the vegetables are tender. Remove at least 2 cups of the beans and vegetables and purée in a blender or food processor. Return the purée to the soup and add the butter; mix well and serve. Serves 8-10.

SHEPHERDS PIE

1 uncooked BROWN RICE FLOUR PIE CRUST p. 92
  (omit cinnamon, sweetener and vanilla)
6 medium potatoes, diced
2 carrots, diced
2 cups cooked Great Northern beans
½-1 cup MISO GRAVY p. 112
2 cups cooked field peas or black-eyed peas
1 cup cooked lima beans
½ tsp. dried basil
¼ tsp. dried marjoram
¼ cup tamari or ⅓ cup liquid soy protein
A little milk, soy milk or NUT MILK p. 124
2 Tbsp. butter or soy margarine
Sea salt and pepper to taste

Prepare 1 crust and set aside, unbaked. (Freeze the remaining dough for use later or make a FRESH FRUIT PIE p. 85 for dessert.) Steam the diced potatoes and carrots, placing the carrots over to one side, so that some potatoes can be removed later to mash for the topping. Meanwhile, combine the Great Northern beans and gravy in a food processor or blender; process until smooth. Combine the bean mixture in a large bowl with the field peas, lima beans, basil, marjoram and tamari; mix well.

When the potatoes and carrots are tender, remove 2½ cups of potatoes and blend with a little milk, butter, salt and pepper to make a mashed potato topping; set aside. Add the remaining potatoes and carrots to the bean mixture; stir well and pour into the pie crust. Spread the mashed potatoes over the top and bake in a preheated oven at 350°F. for about 45 minutes, until the crust and topping are lightly browned. (This dish can be prepared hours ahead and baked just before serving.) Serves 6-8.

Lentils

LENTIL-NUT LOAF

3 cups cooked lentils, drained
1½ cups chopped nuts (almonds, pecans or walnuts)
1 small onion, chopped or 1 tsp. onion powder
½ cup *each* uncooked oatmeal and bread crumbs
½ tsp. *each* sage and celery seed
1 tsp. sea salt
1 Tbsp. liquid soy protein or tamari
¼ cup cold-pressed oil
1 egg or equivalent egg replacer
½ cup lentil stock or vegetable stock

Mix the ingredients together well. Form into a loaf; bake in an oiled loaf pan for 1 hour at 350°F. Serve with gravy or slice for sandwiches. Makes 1 loaf.

LENTIL SOUP

2 Tbsp. butter or soy margarine or to taste
2 cups lentils
2 quarts hot vegetable stock or water
2 medium potatoes *and* 2 carrots, diced
½ lb. fresh or frozen spinach, chopped
1 Tbsp. chopped fresh parsley
½ tsp. dried basil *and* 1 bay leaf
Sea salt and freshly ground pepper to taste

Set the butter aside. Wash the lentils well and combine with the remaining ingredients in a large pot. Simmer for at least 1 hour until the vegetables are tender. Add the butter and mix well. Serves 8-10.

LENTIL-STUFFED CABBAGE

1 large head cabbage

Stuffing:
2 cups cooked lentils
3 cups cooked BROWN RICE p. 92
1 tsp. dried or 1 Tbsp. minced fresh basil
3 Tbsp. miso (diluted with vegetable or lentil stock)
2 Tbsp. powdered vegetable broth
1 tsp. paprika or ½ sweet red pepper, chopped and sautéed
½ onion, chopped and sautéed
1 cup chopped walnuts

Sauce:
1 pint sour cream or plain yogurt
1 cup vegetable stock

1 tsp. paprika
1 tsp. dill
1 Tbsp. tamari or to taste

Wash and core the cabbage; place in a large pot and steam until the leaves are tender and can be easily pulled off the head. Cool and separate the leaves; set aside. Combine all the stuffing ingredients in a large bowl and mix well; place a couple of tablespoonsful on each leaf toward the stem. Then fold over each side and roll toward the leafy edge. Place the stuffed leaves, seam down, in a large, oiled baking dish. Sprinkle with tamari and set aside. Combine all the sauce ingredients and blend well; pour over the stuffed leaves and bake at 350°F for 30 minutes. Serves 8.

Peas

BLACK-EYED PEA SALAD

½ cup chopped celery
½ cup chopped green pepper
½ cup sliced green onions
1 medium-sized hot pepper, chopped
4 cups cooked black-eyed peas
1 large tomato, coarsely chopped
LEMON MISO DRESSING p. 112 or Italian dressing

In a large bowl, combine all the ingredients and mix well. Chill for at least 1 hour (the longer, the better!). Adjust the seasoning and serve on a bed of lettuce or sprouts with a garnish of fresh parsley. Serves 6-8.

FIELD PEAS AND OKRA

2 cups field peas
1 lb. fresh okra, cut into 1-inch lengths

2 Tbsp. butter or soy margarine
½ cup steaming water
Sea salt and freshly ground pepper to taste

Cook the field peas and set aside. Steam the okra for about 5 minutes, until tender; add to the peas. Reserve a little of the steaming water and stir in the butter, if desired, and a little salt and pepper. Add to the peas and okra and toss to coat. Serve immediately in a heated bowl. Serves 4.

GREEN PEAS AND PIGNOLI NUTS

3 Tbsp. pignoli nuts (pine nuts)
3 Tbsp. dry white wine
1 carrot, diced
3 cups fresh peas, shelled
½ tsp. dried or 1 tsp. fresh basil, minced
2 tsp. dried or 1 Tbsp. fresh parsley, minced
2 Tbsp. butter or soy margarine, optional
1 tsp. powdered vegetable broth

Combine the pignoli nuts and wine; set aside. Steam the peas and carrots until tender, about 30 minutes. Combine with the herbs, pignoli nuts and a little of the steaming water in a saucepan; add the butter and powdered broth and mix well. Simmer 5 minutes more to blend the flavors. Serve immediately. Serves 4.

SNOW PEA STIR-FRY

12 dried black mushrooms
1 Tbsp. safflower oil
¾ lb. snow peas
6-8 water chestnuts and 2 small cucumbers
1-2 tsp. toasted sesame oil and 2 Tbsp. tamari

Cut the stems from the black mushrooms; soak in

boiling water for 30 minutes. Drain and slice in half; reserve ½ cup liquid. Wash and string the snow peas and slice the water chestnuts; peel the cucumber and cut into thin 2-inch strips. Heat the safflower oil in a wok or heavy skillet on high. Add the vegetables and stir-fry for 2-3 minutes. Add the sesame oil, tamari and mushroom liquid and toss until the vegetables are tender. Serve immediately with rice. Serves 6.

SPLIT PEA SOUP

2 pkg. dried split peas
3 quarts vegetable stock or water
3 carrots, cut into 1-inch pieces
3-4 medium potatoes, cut into quarters
1 medium onion, optional
¼ cup butter or soy margarine
⅛ tsp. dried basil (or dill or oregano, if preferred)
Sea salt and freshly ground pepper to taste

In Crock Pot: Wash the peas well, carefully removing any stones, and place in a crock pot. Add the vegetable stock, potatoes, carrots, onion and basil. Cook on low heat overnight or all day. About 20 minutes before serving, remove the vegetables and blend them in a food processor until smooth. Return the purée to the soup and add the butter, salt and pepper; thin with more vegetable stock, if necessary. Simmer another 15 minutes and serve with homemade croutons.

In Large Soup Pot: Wash the peas, carefully removing any stones, and place in the pot. Add the vegetable stock and bring to a rolling boil; cut off heat and let soak for at least 1 hour. Add the potatoes, carrots, onion and seasonings; simmer until the peas are thick and 'mushy'. About 15 minutes before serving, remove the vegetables; purée them in a food processor or blender, then return to the soup pot. Add the butter, salt and pepper and thin with more vegetable stock, if necessary. Simmer for 15 more minutes and serve with homemade croutons. Serves 8-10.

Soy Bean Products

Miso

LEMON MISO DRESSING

1 cup plain yogurt
$\frac{1}{4}$ cup white miso
2 tsp. prepared mustard
1 tsp. prepared horseradish
$\frac{1}{4}$ cup olive oil
2 Tbsp. lemon juice
1 tsp. grated lemon peel
White pepper to taste

Combine all the ingredients in a small mixing bowl and whisk until smooth. Serve over your favorite salad greens. Makes $2\frac{1}{2}$ cups.

MISO GRAVY

2 Tbsp. butter or soy margarine
$\frac{1}{3}$ cup rice flour
3 cups vegetable stock
$\frac{1}{4}$ tsp. dried or $\frac{1}{2}$ tsp. chopped fresh basil
$\frac{1}{8}$ tsp. dried or $\frac{1}{4}$ tsp. chopped fresh marjoram
$\frac{1}{4}$ cup miso

Melt the butter in a small saucepan; stir in the flour to make a paste. Slowly add the vegetable stock and herbs, stirring continuously, until thickened; remove from the heat. Dissolve the miso in a small amount of the gravy;

then return to the soup and serve over burgers, nut loaves or rice. Makes 3 cups.

MISO SOUP WITH TOFU NOODLES

¼ lb. (4 oz.) tofu
4 cups vegetable stock
½ cup thinly sliced carrots
1 cup thinly sliced mushrooms
2 cups chopped fresh spinach
¼ cup sliced green onions, optional
¼ tsp. each ground ginger root and cayenne pepper
¼ cup miso

Cut the tofu into very thin (and ¼-inch wide) 'noodles' and set aside. Bring the stock to a boil and prepare the vegetables. Simmer the vegetables and ginger for 5 minutes. Add the tofu and simmer another 2-3 minutes; remove from the heat. Dissolve the miso in a little of the broth; then stir back into the soup. Serve immediately. Serves 4.

Textured Vegetable Protein (Soy Granules)

ANDREA'S VEGETARIAN CHILI

2 Tbsp. cold-pressed oil
1½ cups chopped celery
1½ cups chopped green pepper
1 cup chopped onion
1 clove garlic, minced, optional
8 cups chopped fresh tomatoes or 2 28-oz. cans tomatoes, chopped
6 cups red kidney beans
¼ cup cider or rice vinegar
2 Tbsp. chili powder (more to taste)

2 Tbsp. chopped fresh parsley
2 tsp. sea salt
1½ tsp. dried or 1 Tbsp. fresh basil
1 tsp. dried or 2 tsp. fresh oregano
1½ tsp. ground cumin
¼ tsp. freshly ground pepper
¼ tsp. cayenne pepper, optional
1 bay leaf
¼ cup butter or soy margarine
1 cup textured vegetable protein (soy granules)

In a large pot, sauté the celery, pepper, onion and garlic in the oil until tender. Stir in the remaining ingredients and simmer for 1½ hours. Serve with rice. (It's even better the next day, so prepare ahead, if possible.) Serves 8 with leftovers.

LASAGNA

1 pkg. lasagna noodles (Jerusalem artichoke or whole wheat noodles) or BROWN RICE p. 92
TOFU 'RICOTTA CHEESE' p. 119
MUSHROOM-SOY PASTA SAUCE (below)

Cook the lasagna noodles as directed on the package. Oil a large baking dish and layer the noodles, 'cheese' and sauce. (Brown rice can be layered in place of the noodles.) Repeat the layering until the dish is filled. Bake at 350°F. about 30 minutes until the sauce bubbles. Serves 8.

MUSHROOM-SOY PASTA SAUCE

1 large onion, chopped
2 garlic cloves, minced
½ lb. mushrooms, sliced
¼ cup butter or soy margarine
2 28-oz. cans tomato purée

½ tsp. dried basil
¼ tsp. *each* dried oregano, thyme, and marjoram
1 cup textured vegetable protein
Tamari or sea salt and pepper to taste

In a large pot, sauté the onions, garlic and mushrooms in the butter. Add the tomato purée and herbs; mix well. Stir in the soy granules, tamari or sea salt and pepper; simmer for 30 minutes. Serve over spaghetti, LASAGNA p. 114 or steamed vegetables. (Double the recipe and freeze half for a quick meal later.) Makes 2 quarts.

Tofu

GRILLED 'CHEESE'

⅓ cup white miso
½ tsp. toasted sesame oil
2 Tbsp. cold-pressed oil
2 Tbsp. tahini
1 tsp. minced fresh parsley
1 lb. tofu (firm block)

Combine the miso, oils and tahini; mix well, stir in the parsley and set aside. Slice the tofu into at least 8 slices (thin but as wide as the block) and dry each slice. Spread the miso mixture on top of each tofu slice and place on an oiled cookie sheet. Broil in a preheated oven until lightly browned, about 10 minutes. Turn over and spread the undersides with the remaining miso mixture; broil again until golden brown. Serve on toast or with rice and a salad. Serves 8.

PIZZA SUPREME

Crust:
TOFU BURGER recipe p. 116

Oil 2 pie plates (or muffin tins for mini pizzas) and shape the tofu mixture into crusts about ½-inch thick. Bake at 350°F. for about 35-40 minutes until golden brown and firm to the touch.

Sauce:
2 28-oz. cans tomatoes or 4 lbs. fresh tomatoes
⅛ tsp. garlic powder
1 tsp. mixed Italian herbs
¼ cup butter or soy margarine
Tamari, cooking wine, and pepper to taste

In a large saucepan, combine all the ingredients, except the butter and simmer for at least 1 hour. (Cook half of a fresh carrot in the sauce to remove any bitterness.) Makes 1½ quarts.

Topping:
1 lb. fresh mushrooms, sliced
3 yellow or zucchini squash, sliced
2 cups mung bean sprouts, optional
Sea salt or herb seasoning salt to taste
Grated mild, white, rennetless cheese, optional

In a large skillet, sauté the mushrooms and squash in vegetable oil until tender-crisp; season to taste. Cover the bottom of the precooked crusts with the sauce and layer with the sautéed vegetables. Top with the grated cheese and sprouts, if desired, and bake at 350°F. about 20 minutes to blend the flavors and melt the cheese. Makes two 9-inch pizzas or 24 mini pizzas.

TOFU BURGERS

2 lb. tofu
½ cup chopped green onions, optional
½ lb. carrots, grated
½-1 cup hot taco sauce

¼ tsp. dried basil
½-1 tsp. sea salt
1 cup finely chopped roasted peanuts
¼ cup chopped fresh parsley
1 egg or equivalent egg replacer
1 cup brown rice flour

In a large mixing bowl, crumble the tofu and set aside. Sauté the onions in a little oil and add to the tofu. Add the remaining ingredients and mix very well. Form into patties and fry until browned and crisp on both sides, or bake at 350°F. until firm and browned, about 30 minutes. Makes about 12 burgers.

TOFU-CAROB CREME PUDDING

1 ripe banana
1 lb. tofu, crumbled
½ cup CASHEW CREAM p. 123 or plain yogurt
⅓-½ cup maple syrup
1 tsp. vanilla extract
⅛ tsp. *each* nutmeg and sea salt
¼ cup *each* carob powder and grated coconut

Combine all the ingredients except the coconut in a blender or food processor and blend to a smooth pudding consistency. Pour into a serving dish or individual custard cups and sprinkle with the coconut. Serve as is or chilled. Serves 4.

TOFU CHEESECAKE

Crust: 1 BROWN RICE FLOUR PIE CRUST p. 92, baked

Filling:
1½ lb. tofu
½ cup NUT MILK (almond) p. 124
½ cup maple syrup

1 tsp. vanilla extract
¼ tsp. almond extract
1 Tbsp. lemon juice

Combine all the ingredients in a blender or food processor and blend until smooth. Pour into the crust and bake in a preheated oven at 325°F. for 30 minutes.

Topping:
1 cup dried apricots
2 cups apple juice or apricot nectar
½ cup raisins
¼ tsp. ground cinnamon
¼ cup shredded, unsweetened coconut

Combine all the ingredients in a saucepan and simmer for 30 minutes. Cool and place in a blender or food processor; blend until smooth. Pour as a topping over the tofu filling; chill well before serving. Serves 8.

TOFU EGG(LESS) SALAD

1 lb. tofu
3 Tbsp. Dijon-style mustard
3 Tbsp. diced sweet red pepper
8-10 green olives, chopped
⅓ cup TOFU MAYONNAISE (below)
2 green onions, chopped, optional
2-3 stalks celery, chopped
1 tsp. herb seasoning salt or ½ tsp. sea salt
Freshly ground pepper to taste

Crumble the tofu; add the remaining ingredients and mix well. Serve as a tomato stuffing, a dip for crackers or in pita bread with lettuce and tomato. Serves 4.

TOFU MAYONNAISE

1 lb. tofu

⅓ cup cold-pressed oil
⅓ cup lemon juice
½ tsp. onion powder
½ tsp. dry mustard
1 tsp. herb seasoning salt or ½ tsp. sea salt
⅛ tsp. garlic powder or to taste
1 tsp. apple juice concentrate
(Italian herbs to taste for variety)

Blend the tofu in a food processor until smooth; add the oil, lemon juice and seasonings and blend. Add more oil or lemon juice or a little water to adjust the consistency. Makes about 2½ cups.

TOFU 'RICOTTA CHEESE'

1 lb. tofu
2 Tbsp. cold-pressed oil
¼ cup *each* lemon juice and dried basil
1 tsp. Italian herbs
⅛ tsp. garlic powder, optional
3 green onions, chopped, optional
2 tsp. chopped fresh or 1 tsp. dried parsley
1 tsp. powdered vegetable broth
½ tsp. sea salt or to taste

Blend the tofu in a food processor until creamy, *or* finely crumble the tofu in a bowl. Add the oil, lemon juice, herbs, green onions and salt; mix well. Use in LASAGNA p. 114, manicotti, etc. Makes about 2½ cups.

TOFU-WALNUT BURGERS

Juice of 1 lemon
1 Tbsp. arrowroot
2 Tbsp. miso
1 cup *each* finely chopped celery and walnuts
2 cups cooked BROWN RICE p. 92

½ cup toasted bread crumbs
1 lb. crumbled tofu
½ tsp. *each* sea salt and marjoram
1 tsp. *each* dried basil and grated lemon peel
¼ cup vegetable stock, if needed to moisten

Dissolve the arrowroot in the lemon juice and stir in the miso; set aside. Combine the remaining ingredients in a mixing bowl and knead well. Slowly add the vegetable stock, if too dry. Season to taste and form into patties; place on an oiled baking sheet. Bake in a preheated oven at 350°F. until lightly browned and firm to the touch, about 20 minutes. Makes 8 burgers.

Nuts and seeds

Nuts

ALMOND CREAM

½ cup blanched almonds
½ cup water
2 pitted dates or dried figs
¼ tsp. orange juice concentrate
Pinch of sea salt

In a food processor or blender, chop the almonds to a fine powder; add the remaining ingredients and process until smooth. Serve in place of dairy cream, over fruit, pies or grains. Makes 1 cup.

BANANA-NUT BREAD

4 cups flour (try 2 cups whole wheat, 2 cups unbleached or 1 cup rice flour, 3 cups soy flour)
1 Tbsp. low-sodium baking powder
1 tsp. baking soda

½-1 tsp. sea salt
1 cup melted butter or soy margarine
½ cup apple juice concentrate
¼ cup maple syrup
2 eggs or equivalent egg replacer
5-6 overripe bananas, mashed
½ cup buttermilk
1 Tbsp. cider or rice vinegar
1 cup chopped walnuts
½ cup raisins or currants

Preheat the oven to 350°F. Sift the dry ingredients together; cut in the butter with a pastry blender. Combine the remaining ingredients; stir into the dry mix. Turn into 2 oiled loaf pans and bake for 45-50 minutes or until a toothpick comes out clean. Cool in the pans for 10 minutes, then turn onto a rack. Makes 2 loaves.

BRAZIL NUT BURGERS

½ cup ground Brazil nuts
¼ cup ground sunflower seeds (sunflower meal)
½ cup ground sesame seeds (sesame meal)
1 cup cooked BROWN RICE p. 92
¼ cup brown rice flour
1 egg or equivalent egg replacer
2 tsp. chili powder
1 Tbsp. minced onion, optional
Tamari or herb seasoning salt to taste

Combine all the ingredients and knead into a ball. Form into burgers and brown on both sides in an oiled skillet or bake at 350°F. until lightly browned, about 20 minutes. Makes 8.

CAROB BROWNIES

$\frac{1}{3}$ cup maple syrup
2 Tbsp. blackstrap molasses
$\frac{1}{4}$ cup cold-pressed oil
2 eggs or equivalent egg replacer
1 tsp. vanilla extract
$\frac{1}{2}$ cup *each* rice flour and carob powder
$\frac{1}{2}$ cup finely ground sunflower seeds
$\frac{1}{2}$ tsp. *each* ginger and cinnamon
$\frac{1}{2}$ cup chopped nuts or raisins

Combine the wet ingredients in a large bowl. In another bowl, mix together the dry ingredients; add a little at a time to the wet mixture to make a stiff batter. Stir in the nuts or raisins and turn into an oiled 8-inch pan. Bake at 350°F. for 25 minutes. Cool and cut into squares. Makes 16 brownies.

CAROB-PEANUT BUTTER FUDGE BALLS

$\frac{1}{4}$ cup butter or soy margarine
$\frac{1}{3}$ cup maple syrup
6 Tbsp. carob powder
$\frac{1}{3}$ cup milk or NUT MILK p. 124 (more if needed)
$\frac{1}{2}$-1 cup peanut butter (if unsalted, add $\frac{1}{4}$ tsp. sea salt)
1 tsp. vanilla extract
3 cups oatmeal

In a small saucepan, melt the butter; add the syrup and carob and bring to a boil. Add the milk and simmer for 5 minutes, stirring continuously. Remove from the heat; add the peanut butter and vanilla and mix well. Stir in the oatmeal, 1 cup at a time. Drop by the teaspoonful onto wax paper, cool and serve. Makes 3 dozen balls.

CASHEW CREAM

½ cup cashews
½ cup water
1 Tbsp. sweetener (maple syrup, apple juice concentrate, rice syrup or 2 pieces of dried fruit)
¼ tsp. vanilla extract
Pinch of sea salt

In a food processor or blender, chop the cashews to a fine powder; add the remaining ingredients and process until smooth. Serve as you would dairy cream, over fruit, pies or grains. Makes 1 cup.

COCONUT MACAROONS

2 Tbsp. maple syrup
¼ cup cashew butter or tahini
Pinch of sea salt
¼ tsp. vanilla extract
2 Tbsp. chopped pecans
1 cup shredded unsweetened coconut
Extra coconut for rolling

Blend the maple syrup, cashew butter or tahini, salt and vanilla together well (add a couple of Tbsp. water if too thick). Stir in the pecans, then the coconut. Form into small balls and roll in the extra coconut until coated. Chill and serve unbaked or bake at 350°F. for 15 minutes, until lightly browned. Makes 1½ dozen small balls.

NUT BUTTER

2 cups raw or lightly toasted nuts (cashews, blanched almonds or peanuts)
Sea salt to taste, optional

Place the nuts in a food processor or grinder and process

to the desired consistency. (The longer the processing the more oil is released.) Add salt if desired, blend again. Makes about 1½ cups.

NUT MILK

1 cup nuts (blanched almonds, cashews, pecans, etc.)
3 cups water

Chop the nuts in a blender or food processor until finely powdered; add the water and blend for 3 minutes. Strain, if desired, and reserve the nut pulp for cereal or baking. Serve hot or cold. Makes 1 quart.

Note: when serving NUT MILK as a beverage or with cereal, etc. add:

2 tsp. sweetener (barley malt, carob, rice syrup, maple syrup or apple juice concentrate)
1 tsp. vanilla extract

PEANUT BUTTER COOKIES

¼ cup butter or soy margarine, melted
¼-½ cup maple syrup
1 egg or equivalent egg replacer
1 cup peanut butter
½ tsp. vanilla extract
1 Tbsp. cider or rice vinegar
½ tsp. sea salt (if unsalted peanut butter is used)
½ tsp. baking soda
2 cups soy flour

Preheat the oven to 375°F. In a large mixing bowl, combine the wet ingredients and beat until smooth. Sift in the dry ingredients and mix well. Roll the dough into 1-inch balls and place on an oiled cookie sheet; flatten with a fork and bake for about 15 minutes. Makes about 2 dozen cookies.

PEANUT BUTTER SOUP

1 medium onion, chopped
1 cup chopped celery
2 Tbsp. cold-pressed oil
¼ cup peanut butter
1½ cups vegetable stock *and* 2 cups tomato juice
½ tsp. ground coriander
⅛ tsp. ground white pepper and sea salt to taste
1 tsp. powdered vegetable broth
Plain yogurt, optional

In a large saucepan, sauté the onion and celery in the oil until tender. Stir in the peanut butter; add the vegetable stock, tomato juice and seasonings. Bring to a boil and simmer for 10 minutes. Serve in individual bowls, topped with a spoonful of yogurt. Serves 4.

PLUSH PECAN PIE

Crust: 1 GRANOLA pie crust p. 89, baked

Filling:
¼ cup quick-cooking, granulated tapioca
1 cup apple juice
¼ cup maple syrup
¼ cup butter or soy margarine
1 tsp. vanilla extract
2 cups pecan halves or pieces

Heat the tapioca and apple juice in a saucepan, stirring continuously, for about 5 minutes. Add the maple syrup and butter, stirring until the butter is melted. Stir in the vanilla and pecans. Pour into the crust; bake at 350°F. for 20 minutes. Cool and serve. Serves 8.

WALNUT PATTIES

1 cup chopped walnuts

½ cup ground sunflower seeds
1 cup grated carrots
½ cup minced celery
1 cup oatmeal
1 Tbsp. cold-pressed oil
2 Tbsp. finely chopped onion, optional
Pinch of sage
Tamari or herb seasoning salt to taste
Vegetable stock, as needed

Mix all the ingredients together well in a large mixing bowl. Form into patties and brown on both sides in an oiled skillet or bake at 350°F. until browned, about 20 minutes. Makes 8 patties.

Seeds

PUMPKIN SEED CRACKERS

¼ cup ground pumpkin seeds
½ cup *each* rice flour and oat flour
1-2 Tbsp. sesame oil
⅛ tsp. sea salt or herb seasoning salt

Combine all the ingredients and knead into a ball. Roll out about ¼-inch thick on waxed paper and cut into circles. Place on a cookie sheet and bake at 350°F. for about 5-10 minutes until lightly browned. Makes about 2 dozen.

SESAME CANDY

2 Tbsp. sesame oil
1-2 Tbsp. maple syrup
Pinch of sea salt
2 drops vanilla extract
1 cup ground sesame seeds

2 Tbsp. ground almonds

Blend together the oil, syrup, salt and vanilla. Stir in the ground seeds and almonds until thoroughly mixed. Form the mixture into a thin roll and chill. Slice when ready to serve. Makes about $1\frac{1}{2}$ dozen slices.

SESAME HALVAH

1 cup tahini (or sesame butter)
Maple syrup to taste

Stir the tahini until creamy (so the oil is well mixed with the pulp). Add the maple syrup slowly while stirring, until the mixture becomes thick and crumbly and as sweet as desired. Serve on crackers, biscuits, or a sweet bread (challah).

SUNFLOWER SEED ROLL

1 cup ground sunflower seeds
$\frac{1}{4}$ cup chopped nuts
$\frac{1}{2}$ cup chopped dried fruit (raisins, dates, apricots, apples, etc.)
1 Tbsp. maple syrup or fruit juice concentrate
$\frac{1}{8}$ tsp. vanilla extract
Pinch of sea salt
$\frac{1}{4}$ cup nut butter (e.g., cashew, almond, tahini, peanut)

Blend all the ingredients together well. Knead into a ball and form into a roll. Chill and slice when ready to serve. (Or flatten the kneaded ball to $\frac{1}{2}$-inch thickness on a buttered platter; chill and cut into squares.) Makes about 2 dozen pieces.

SUPER SNACK

$\frac{1}{4}$ cup *each* cashews, almonds and peanuts
$\frac{1}{4}$ cup *each* sesame, sunflower and pumpkin seeds

Combine the nuts and seeds and toast lightly or serve raw. Sprinkle with a little herb seasoning salt, if desired, and keep on hand for a snack. Makes 1½ cups.

Vegetables

ASPARAGUS-PASTA SALAD

1½-2 lb. fresh asparagus
12 cherry tomatoes, quartered
1 cup sliced black olives
½ cup pignoli nuts (pine nuts)
3 Tbsp. fresh minced parsley
10 oz. spaghetti (rice spaghetti, if available)
¼ cup rice vinegar
¼ cup lemon juice
½ cup olive oil
2 tsp. dried oregano
1 tsp. dried marjoram
1 tsp. powdered vegetable broth
Herb seasoning salt and freshly ground pepper to taste

To prepare the asparagus for cooking: hold the stem and the tip ends between the fingertips of each hand. Bend the asparagus until it breaks. Discard the stem ends, cut the tip ends into 1-inch pieces and steam until tender-crisp. Combine the steamed asparagus, tomatoes, olives, pignoli nuts and parsley in a large mixing bowl and set aside. Cook the rice spaghetti; drain and rinse with cold water. Add to the asparagus mixture. In a screw-top jar, combine the remaining ingredients and shake well; pour over the vegetables and pasta and toss. Adjust the seasoning and chill well before serving. Serves 8.

BEETS WITH LEMON-GINGER SAUCE

12 small beets
1 tsp. ground ginger or 2 tsp. grated fresh ginger
¾ cup LEMON MISO DRESSING p. 112

Wash the beets (leave the skin, the root end and about 1 inch of the stem to help retain the color while cooking). Place in a steamer in a large saucepan and cover tightly. Steam until just tender, about 30 minutes. Then run cold water over the beets; peel off the skins, trim the roots and stems and slice. Mix the ginger with the dressing and stir with the beets. Serve hot or cold. Serves 4.

BROCCOLI HOLLANDAISE

1 large head broccoli
3 Tbsp. butter or soy margarine
3 Tbsp. rice flour
1½ cups NUT MILK (cashew) p. 124
⅓ cup lemon juice
⅛ tsp. cayenne pepper (more to taste)
Sea salt to taste

Break or cut the broccoli into bite-sized pieces and steam until tender-crisp. Meanwhile, prepare the 'hollandaise' sauce: melt the butter in a medium-sized saucepan on low heat. Add the flour and mix well. Slowly add the cashew milk, stirring until the mixture is quite thick and creamy. Remove from the heat. Add the lemon juice, cayenne pepper and salt; mix well. Place the steamed broccoli in a heated serving dish, cover with the sauce and serve. Serves 6-8.

BRUSSELS SPROUTS SALAD

1 lb. Brussels sprouts
1 Tbsp. fresh parsley, minced

¼ cup fresh lemon juice
2 Tbsp. olive oil
1 tsp. grated lemon peel
1 Tbsp. apple juice concentrate
Herb seasoning salt and white pepper to taste

Rinse and trim the Brussels sprouts; soak in cold water for 20-30 minutes and drain. Steam until just tender, 15-20 minutes. Remove and set aside to cool. Meanwhile, combine the remaining ingredients in a screw-top jar; shake well and pour over the cooled sprouts. Chill well before serving on a bed of lettuce. Serves 4.

CABBAGE AND APPLES

2 Tbsp. butter or soy margarine
½ cup onion, cut in rings
6 cups shredded red cabbage
¼ cup lemon juice
¼ tsp. sea salt
½ tsp. *each* ground cinnamon and nutmeg
½ tsp. *each* cardamom or allspice and fennel seeds
3 apples, cored and sliced
¼ cup *each* apple juice concentrate and orange juice
¼ cup chopped walnuts

Melt the butter in a large skillet; sauté the onion, add the cabbage and cover. Simmer for 5-10 minutes, until almost tender. Stir in the lemon juice, salt and spices. In a large casserole, layer the cabbage and apple slices, several layers deep. Mix the apple and orange juice concentrates and pour over the top. Cover and bake at 375°F. for about 30 minutes. Serves 4-6.

CARROT BAKE

3 cups grated carrots
3 Tbsp. butter or soy margarine

Sea salt and freshly ground pepper to taste
Pinch of cinnamon, optional

Bake the grated carrots in a tightly covered 1-quart casserole dish at 325°F. for 30 minutes. (Do not add water.) Remove from the oven, add the butter and seasonings and serve immediately. Serves 6.

CAULIFLOWER CURRY

1 head fresh cauliflower
4 Tbsp. butter or soy margarine
1 tsp. salt or tamari
1 large onion, finely chopped
½ cup dried red lentils or 1 cup cooked brown lentils, drained
¾ tsp. chili powder
¼ tsp. turmeric
¾ tsp. curry powder
3 Tbsp. dried grated coconut
1 cup water
Juice of 1 lemon

Break the cauliflower into bite-sized pieces; set aside. In a large skillet, sauté the onions in the butter until tender. Add the cauliflower and the remaining ingredients except the lemon juice. Cook on low heat until tender, about 30 minutes. Then add the lemon juice, adjust the seasoning and serve. Serves 4-6.

CELERY BAKE

1 whole head celery, washed
1 Tbsp. cold-pressed oil
1 tsp. sesame oil
1 Tbsp. lemon juice
1 Tbsp. tamari
6 green onions, chopped

Place the oil and the whole celery head in the bottom of a covered baking dish. Sprinkle the lemon juice and tamari over the celery; cover and bake at 350°F. for 30 minutes. Add the green onions to the celery and bake for another 15 minutes. Serves 4.

CUCUMBER MOUSSE

4 Tbsp. agar-agar flakes
1 cup vegetable stock or water
1 cup TOFU MAYONNAISE p. 118
1 Tbsp. sliced green onions
1 Tbsp. lemon juice
½ tsp. dried dill
⅛ tsp. garlic powder
Sea salt and bottled hot sauce to taste
2 medium cucumbers, peeled

In a small saucepan, bring the agar-agar and vegetable stock to a boil; simmer for about 5 minutes, stirring continuously. Stir in the mayonnaise, green onion, lemon juice, dill, garlic, salt and hot sauce; set aside to cool. Purée the cucumber in a food processor or blender and add the cooled agar mixture; blend until smooth. Pour into a 5-cup mold and chill until firm, about 4 hours. Unmold onto a lettuce-lined plate; garnish with radish roses and fresh parsley. Serves 8.

GREENS (KALE, TURNIP OR COLLARD GREENS)

4 lb. fresh greens, washed and chopped
1-2 Tbsp. butter or soy margarine, optional
3 Tbsp. powdered vegetable broth
1 tsp. herb seasoning salt or ½ tsp. sea salt
1-2 Tbsp. lemon juice

Steam the greens until tender, about 15 minutes. Add the remaining ingredients, mix well and place in a heated serving bowl. (If fresh greens are not available, frozen may be substituted.) Serves 6.

JERUSALEM ARTICHOKES WITH GINGER BUTTER

1 lb. fresh Jerusalem artichokes, cut bite-sized
2 Tbsp. grated fresh ginger
2 Tbsp. butter or soy margarine
1 tsp. powdered vegetable broth

Steam the artichokes until just tender. Melt the butter in a small saucepan and sauté the ginger; stir in the powdered vegetable broth (dilute with vegetable stock if needed). Add the steamed artichokes and toss gently; serve immediately. Serves 4-6.

MUSHROOMS WITH NUT STUFFING

3 lb. giant mushrooms
3 stalks celery, chopped
1 small onion, chopped
1 cup pecans (or other nuts), chopped
1 can water chestnuts, chopped
3½ cups breadcrumbs (10 slices, whole grain toast)
¼ cup butter or soy margarine
⅛ tsp. dried basil and/or tarragon
Herb seasoning salt or sea salt and pepper to taste

Clean the mushrooms and chop the stems to use in the stuffing. In a large mixing bowl, combine the chopped stems and the remaining ingredients; mix well. Arrange the mushroom caps in an oiled baking pan. Fill with the stuffing mixture and bake about 15 minutes at 350°F., then broil for 5 minutes. Makes 2-3 dozen.

OKRA STEW

¼ cup cold-pressed oil

¼ cup chopped onions, optional
1 cup chopped celery
1 cup diced sweet red pepper
2 cups thinly sliced okra
2 cups chopped fresh tomatoes
1 cup vegetable stock or water
Sea salt and cayenne pepper to taste

Sauté the onions, celery and peppers in the oil until tender; add the remaining ingredients. Simmer for 30 minutes; season to taste and serve with rice. Serves 8.

PARSNIPS AND CARROTS

½ lb. carrots, cut into julienne strips
½ lb. parsnips, cut into julienne strips
¼ cup plain yogurt
1 Tbsp. fresh parsley, minced
2 tsp. minced fresh dill or 1 tsp. dried dill
2 Tbsp. butter or soy margarine (skip this step if serving cold as a salad)
Sea salt and freshly ground pepper to taste

Steam the carrots for about 5 minutes; add the parsnips and steam until tender. Combine the remaining ingredients and set aside. When the vegetables are cooked, drain and stir in the yogurt mixture. Serve hot or cold. Serves 4.

SPINACH-MUSHROOM BAKE

1 lb. fresh spinach, chopped
1 lb. fresh mushrooms, sliced
1 cup TOFU 'RICOTTA CHEESE' p. 119
1 Tbsp. butter or soy margarine
¼ tsp. garlic powder
Sea salt and freshly ground pepper to taste
3 Tbsp. Italian-seasoned bread crumbs for garnish

In a large saucepan, sauté the mushrooms in butter until tender. Add the spinach, cover and cook for 3 minutes; add the remaining ingredients. Mix well; pour into an oiled casserole dish and top with bread crumbs. Bake at 350°F. about 20 minutes. Serves 4-6.

Squash

ACORN SQUASH AND APPLES

2 medium-sized acorn squash
2 apples
1 cup apple juice
½ tsp. *each* ground cinnamon and sea salt
½ cup chopped pecans
Butter or soy margarine

Bake the squash whole at 375°F. for 1 hour or until soft. Remove from the oven and set aside to cool. Meanwhile, core and finely chop the apples; place in a saucepan with the apple juice, cinnamon and salt and simmer until tender. When the squash has cooled, cut each squash in half. Remove the seeds, scoop out the meat and add with the pecans to the apple mixture. Mash all together well and place in a baking dish; dot with butter and broil until lightly browned. Serves 4.

BUTTERNUT SQUASH WITH CARROT STUFFING

2 small butternut squash
1 cup grated carrots
¼ cup raisins
¼ cup orange juice
Pinch of cinnamon, optional
4 tsp. butter or soy margarine

Cut the butternut squash into halves, remove the seeds

and set aside. Combine the carrots, raisins, juice and cinnamon; stuff into the squash centers. Place in a baking pan and dot with butter. Bake at 350°F. for 40 minutes, or until tender. Serves 4.

SPAGHETTI SQUASH

Place 1 large spaghetti squash on an oiled baking dish; bake at 350°F. for 1 hour or until tender. Cut the squash in half lengthwise and scoop out the seeds. Then empty the shells with a fork, gently pulling out the spaghetti-like squash threads. If the threads do not come out easily, turn each half over in a baking dish with a little water and bake 15-20 minutes longer. Serve with tomato sauce, or a sauce of melted butter and summer savory or mix with TOFU 'RICOTTA CHEESE' p. 119 and MUSHROOM-SOY PASTA SAUCE p. 114 in a casserole. Serves 8.

YELLOW SQUASH

2 lb. yellow squash, thinly sliced
1 medium onion, thinly sliced, optional
Herb seasoning salt or sea salt and pepper to taste
Summer savory, optional
2 Tbsp. butter or soy margarine

Steam the sliced squash (and onion) until tender-crisp, about 15 minutes. Melt the butter in a little of the water from the steaming and stir in the seasonings. Pour over the squash and serve immediately. Serves 8.

ZUCCHINI OREGANO

Cut 4 medium zucchini in half lengthwise. Steam for about 12-15 minutes or until tender. Scoop out the centers and mix with butter and oregano. Refill the shells. Sprinkle with Parmesan cheese and broil for 5-10 minutes to brown lightly. Serves 8.